Manage Your
Life
Before Life
Manages You

Published in 2015
Printed in the United States of America
Library of Congress Control Number:
Print: ISBN 978-0-9797958-2-4
E-Book: ISBN 978-0-9797958-1-7

Book design by Stacey Aaronson

Sophia Press
Annapolis, MD
www.aliciamrodriguez.com

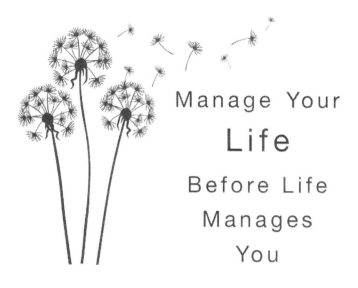

Manage Your
Life
Before Life
Manages
You

More Joy and Less Stress
in 365 Days

By
Alicia M. Rodriguez

Sophia Press

This book is dedicated to my readers, those of you who know that joy and harmony can go hand in hand with a successful and fulfilling life. This book is meant to inspire you, and to teach you to inspire yourself.

INTRODUCTION

What would it be like to choose each day, instead of waking up each morning to habitual patterns that rob you of your vitality, your joy, and, ultimately, your life force? How would your life be different if each day you created the container for a high-quality existence?

For years I have coached thousands of individuals in all walks of life, from CEOs and nonprofit executives to young professionals, artists, and entrepreneurs. Not one has ever said, "I wish my life were more stressful." As life gets faster and more complex, people are striving to find more peace and harmony amid its demands. Yet still they find themselves losing touch with what really matters, until some catalyst appears to wake them from their trance.

Each day is an opportunity to make a slight change in your thinking, your actions, and your feelings. When you make changes one day at a time, you will soon find that your entire life begins to shift. I often say to my clients who want to make transitions in their life, "Just do one thing differently today. Just one thing." And with that, they find that changes occur effortlessly.

Maybe it's a change in the way you wake up each morning. Maybe it's taking a five-minute breathing break between meetings. Maybe it's driving in silence, instead of making phone calls. These are just small, easy-to-make adjustments that cumulatively have a positive effect on the quality of your life.

There are no big action plans, accountability sessions, or to-do lists in this book. Over the next 365 days, you will be inspired to make the changes you need to successfully manage your life. Supported by reflective questions and simple exercises, you will begin to feel refreshed and renewed, will begin to live in alignment with what matters most to you, and will experience more joy and ease. That vitality will show up in your work, in your relationships, and in your increased self-confidence.

Begin now to manage your life before life manages you. It will require a daily intention and a commitment to doing things differently. Take time each day to reflect on the questions I ask you. Write down your thoughts and inquiries, make doodles, and scribble to your heart's content on any and all of these pages. Use a journal if you'd like. Engage! Start actively participating in your life! And have fun while you create more harmony and joy.

After 365 days, be sure to celebrate. And start over again. Life is movement, dynamic and ever changing. Be present in the flow of your life from this day forward. It's your life. Now own it.

Warmest wishes,

Alicia

— DAY 1 —

CHECK IN WITH YOURSELF

Today, ask yourself, "Who am I?" Are you really happy right now in your life, or are you uncomfortable? Do you sense that something needs to change, without knowing what it is? Today you'll check in with yourself for the purpose of connecting with a deep appreciation for your life. Coming up over the next ten days: ten elements to consider as you shift from stress to joy.

— DAY 2 —

ELEMENT #1: CREATE STILLNESS

Consciously create still (mental, emotional, physical, spiritual) space in your life. You could meditate, go for quiet walks in nature, begin a yoga practice, or do anything else that quiets your mind and body. I often like to cook or kayak to create stillness. Stillness does not necessarily mean not moving; it could be anything that creates inner peace and openness for you.

— DAY 3 —

ELEMENT #2: GET BACK TO THE EARTH

If you like to garden, get your hands in the dirt, watch your vegetables grow, and bring nourishment to your table. If you like animals, go play with them, watch them, and listen to them. If you love being in nature, spend a day at the beach or take time to walk through woods or go on a gentle hike in the mountains.

— DAY 4 —

ELEMENT #3: VALUE YOUR FRIENDSHIPS

Surround yourself with loving people who value you for who you are, just the way you are: individuals who tell the truth and manifest personal integrity; friends who energize you and challenge you to be the very best you.

— DAY 5 —

ELEMENT #4: BE TRUE TO YOUR BEST SELF

Don't ever make the mistake of allowing others to tell you who you are supposed to be. You are who *you* choose to be and say you are, and no one can tell you differently. On this page or in your journal, make two columns. In column one, write: "Up Until Now." In column two, write: "From This Point On." Complete each column, based on the following example: "Up until now, I have been timid. From this point on, I will be courageous in my interactions with others." Revisit this page when you notice that a new story needs to be written about how you present yourself to the world.

— DAY 6 —

ELEMENT #5:
DEVELOP A SPIRITUAL PRACTICE

Explore your own spirituality, be it in the form of a structured religion, a contemplative practice of still-ness, or a prayer before your personal altar. Create daily rituals that allow you to connect to your heart and soul. Connect with the divine, in whatever way you conceive it to exist.

— DAY 7 —

ELEMENT #6: PRACTICE SELF-CARE

Today, honor and nourish your body, heart, and mind. When you feel healthy and well rested, you are better able to remain centered, even in the face of resistance and challenges. You may be inclined to run or swim, or perhaps, like I do, you find kayaking more in line with your desire to nourish yourself physically. Good nutrition feeds the body and promotes well-being, as does a night of delicious sleep. As you begin to reconnect with your essential being, you will begin to notice what works for you. Listen to your intuition and your body for clues to your personal wellness.

— DAY 8 —

ELEMENT #7: IMAGINE THAT YOU HAD ONLY 48 HOURS TO LIVE

What would you do? Whom would you be with? Where would you be? The answers to these questions will point to those values you hold dearest.

Write these answers on this page or in a journal, and begin to change your activities and adjust toward these answers. Record how you feel when you move into alignment with your answers to reinforce the changes you are making.

— DAY 9 —

ELEMENT #8: ASK YOURSELF, "WHO AM I?"

This is a koan (a riddle that cannot be unraveled with the mind) that the Zen masters ask their pupils —and ask, and ask, and ask. Use the koan. Ask yourself this question at least fifty times (really!). Write down the answers, and listen to them; this is an opportunity to learn what is true for you. Explore your answers to see which ones resonate the most with you. Write down your thoughts on how you can align more with these responses.

— DAY 10 —
ELEMENT #9: GET A NEW PERSPECTIVE

Today, you'll do an exercise that will help you see yourself as others see you. Very rarely do we witness our greatness—or our limitations—in the same way others do. We may be blind to the effect we have on others when we are not at our best. Ask people whom you trust for five adjectives that describe you. Do not elaborate on the request. Allow them to give you the gift of reflection. Look for how often the same word comes up. What surprises you? What would you like to embrace about this feedback? What would you like to change about the way you are perceived? Write down your answers.

— DAY 11 —
ELEMENT #10: DEFINE SUCCESS

You may be defining success according to society's measures, when you may not actually believe those measures are right for you at this point. Complete this sentence to begin to understand what success means to you: "I know I am successful when I feel/think/do . . ."

— DAY 12 —
APPLY THE TEN ELEMENTS

Apply the Ten Elements to your work or business as well as to your personal life. Has your business environment been changing since the time you started your business or were hired for your current position? How does your personal evolution impact the changes that may be occurring in your work and vice versa? Incorporate what you are learning about yourself into your future plans for business or career. The Ten Elements help you integrate the dimensions of your life to create wholeness, health and happiness for you.

DAY 13

MOVE WITH THE FLOW OF CHANGE

You may feel that letting go of things of the past is frightening. You may cling to those things for dear life, preferring the known to the unknown. If you are asking yourself, "Who am I?" for the first time in years, you may discover a different answer that will require something unfamiliar, perhaps a transformation of your beliefs. Life is dynamic. Change your approach from *letting go* to *moving with*, and create more ease. When you move with your natural state of being, there will be less resistance, and new possibilities will emerge that support the changes you want to make to better manage your life. If you notice that your health needs attention, start now to incorporate healthy habits into your daily routine. If you notice that your friendships are toxic, start now to cultivate new relationships that support your values. By moving with the flow of your life, you will inevitably move away from what does not serve you.

— DAY 14 —
GET COMFORTABLE WITH THE NEW NORMAL

Where in your life or your work do you default to past behaviors or patterns that used to work for you? Notice whether you are using them as a default because they are known, because they are a comfortable way of being, or because they are a way of doing things that is simply easier for you. Is it time to open yourself up to some discomfort and learn to enlist other aspects of yourself? There are three steps to moving through your discomfort. First, notice the discomfort without judgment. Second, identify what needs to change. Third, intentionally begin to incorporate the change in your life. You will find that taking these three steps will allow you to move through the discomfort and stop defaulting to old behaviors that no longer serve you.

— DAY 15 —
CREATE HARMONY

If you tend to live in your mind, consider how you can use your body to learn. Or if you tend to be highly analytical, how can you exercise the muscle of intuition? How can you use all the gifts and talents you have available to you, not just the ones you are used to using? Begin to incorporate these diminished aspects of yourself into your life. Identifying these imbalances will help you to expand your potential and give you greater access to your endless possibilities.

— DAY 16 —
LIVE ACCORDING TO YOUR TRUTH

Sometimes suddenly, sometimes slowly, your unhappiness and discomfort begin to assert themselves to a point where you can no longer tolerate the feeling that you are not living in accordance with what matters most to you. You realize that you are paying a price for living someone else's version of your life. Once you realize this, you will already be on your way to creating new ways of being. This discomfort is a signal that something needs to change so that you can fulfill your potential. Actively engage the discomfort, use the three steps in Day 14 to move through the discomfort, and incorporate changes gradually.

DAY 17
BEGIN IN THE PRESENT

You can create the future only in the present. Staying stuck in the past will keep you from living your best life now. Worrying about the future will keep you from creating the steps you need to take to better manage your life now. There is only one place to begin. Start now. Read this book daily, and practice your way into a future you desire.

— DAY 18 —
SEEK WHOLENESS

You may tend to polarize your situation by seeing possibilities as mutually exclusive, instead of searching for how you might creatively include multiple aspects of your desired life. For example, you may believe that you have to choose between work and exercise because you don't have time to do both. This attitude sets up work and exercise as mutually exclusive. To shift to a life that includes both, you will find that the key is scheduling time in your day or week to include exercise and perhaps enlisting a friend to join you. You can transform how you perceive your life in ways that fuel your next evolution. Seek integration and wholeness, instead of polarizing your possibilities.

— DAY 19 —
BALANCE THE YIN AND YANG OF YOUR LIFE

To be the person you are is to expand and retreat at the same time. In your external world, you expand who you are by adding new dimensions to your life.

You incorporate new activities and new relationships that support the changes you are making. In your internal world, you retreat to the beginning, to the essential self, the one that dearly wants and needs to be acknowledged and represented, perhaps in new ways that may at first be surprising. You begin a contemplative practice and become more attuned to your inner dialogue, generating feelings of self-worth and confidence and peace and harmony.

– DAY 20 –
APPRECIATE YOUR SELF

Why does your life seem to manage you, instead of the reverse? It's likely that you have been trying to live up to someone else's version of who you are—and creating tension and unease in the process. To be fully the person you are is the only thing your soul demands. You will pay a price for living someone else's life, when living your own, big, perfect, beautiful life is all that you are meant to do. Today, do one thing to appreciate your Self. Buy yourself some flowers, get a massage, call someone you love, or cook yourself a beautiful meal.

— DAY 21 —

IDENTIFY YOUR BOUNDARIES

What is a boundary? Is it a wall you construct to keep others out? Is it solid or permeable? How is a boundary set? Merriam-Webster's online dictionary defines "boundary" as "a line or plane indicating the limit or extent of something, a line determining the limits of an area." Let's consider and reframe these definitions in light of being human. Take a moment and write down what boundaries you are aware of. What are the lines that cannot be crossed? What is unacceptable to you? Jot down your thoughts; in the next few days, we will explore boundaries further.

— DAY 22 —

DEFINE YOUR VALUES

A boundary can be defined as a personal demarcation of values that maintain wholeness and integrity. By that same definition, a boundary is a personal tool that keeps you whole, distinct, alive, supported, and healthy. It is based on values you hold essential to your well-being and happiness.

These values could be time with family, education, hobbies, honesty, work ethic, service, and more. Crossing a boundary can diminish or compromise your wholeness. If you understand what matters to you, then you can more easily define, articulate, and honor your own boundaries. Do you know what your values are now? How are you expressing or not expressing these? Use this page or your journal to record your answers and thoughts.

— DAY 23 —
COMMIT TO POSSIBILITIES

What have been some of your most meaningful experiences over time? What makes them meaningful to you? When you commit to living your life in alignment with what matters most to you, amazing possibilities will arise and setting boundaries will become easier. You will attract relationships based on respect and care, and you will enjoy renewed energy at work. The whining will cease, and in its place you may hear a resounding roar of vitality and joy!

— DAY 24 —
DEVELOP COURAGE

Life is inherently uncertain. The knowledge of this fact keeps you seeking safety and security. Fear keeps you from acting on your deepest desires. The way to cope with that fear is to acknowledge it and develop courage. Courage is what will help you take action toward creating a full and rich life. Where could you be more courageous?

— DAY 25 —
CHECK IN WITH YOURSELF

I have developed a practice of periodically asking myself, "Is this really what I want to be doing right now?" There are times when I say yes, and times when it is crystal clear that I should not be doing what I am doing. We all must do things we do not enjoy, but this is a question that builds a high degree of awareness around where you spend your time and your energy. Practice asking yourself this question. Set an alarm or reminder once or twice a day, and make this question the alarm label. In implementing this practice, you will become more aware of, and intentional about, where your attention and energy are focused.

— DAY 26 —
STOP BLAMING YOURSELF

Blame and shame are insidious and can creep into your thoughts unconsciously. Every experience you have in your life is an opportunity to learn about your essential self. Mistakes identify places that do not align with your highest expression of yourself. Notice them, learn from them, and move on without blame. Forgive yourself for your human condition, and you will become more compassionate toward and forgiving of others. This is an important lesson in creating more joy and less stress in your life.

— DAY 27 —
FULFILL YOUR NEEDS

Everyone has needs. Some needs are fundamental, such as the need to be loved or to be appreciated. Get your needs met before you become resentful. As an example, if you need more quiet time to maintain wellness, build it into your day or week and be explicit about this requirement with anyone with whom you have a relationship. When you do not meet your needs, you project this need onto others and cause more stress and tension. Fulfill your needs before they become overwhelming or result in huge conflict. Meeting your needs first will build a foundation of resilience that allows you to create what you want in your life.

— DAY 28 —
ASK FOR HELP

Whether you want to admit it or not, you need other people to help you succeed. Sometimes you just have to ask for help, regardless of how independent you think you are. Asking for help is not a sign of weakness; it takes courage and confidence to do so. Whom do you need to ask for help in creating a life of joy and less stress? What is your specific request of those people? Be specific, so they can evaluate whether and/or how they can help you.

— DAY 29 —
TAKE RESPONSIBILITY FOR YOUR NEEDS

Ultimately, you are the one responsible for getting your needs met. Don't depend on others to know what these are. Make direct, specific requests, find alternatives, and create structures in your life that position you to have your needs met. When you act with purpose, you open the way for more ease in your life and a better connection to others.

— DAY 30 —
TAKE THE RIGHT ACTION

When you want to achieve something, your natural inclination may be to take action. There are many times when this is exactly what is called for. However, when taking action becomes a knee-jerk reaction to everything, it becomes a pattern of behavior that arises from non-thinking. How powerful would your actions be if they were preceded by a pause, however small, to reflect on the appropriate action to take, or the right words to use, to create space and defuse a potentially volatile situation? By being diligent and precise with your intention, you can create a blueprint that moves you forward toward the outcome you desire. When your energy is more focused, you become more productive.

— DAY 31 —
FIND YOUR RESET BUTTON

Do you run through your day as if you were on a treadmill two notches too high for you? Do you move from one task to another, or from mini-crisis to mini-crisis, without taking a "pause" or a breath for yourself? How does your body feel at the end of the day? If you are noticing these feelings, it's time to find your personal reset button and use it! Here are some simple ways to hit that button when you most need to:

1) Leave time between meetings to review actions to take and to ready your mind to receive new information at the next meeting.

2) When you arrive home from work (or if you work from home, whenever you finish your workday), take thirty minutes to change your clothes, put them away, and downshift from your work pace. This will allow you to be more present to your family, and to experience your evening without tension.

3) Create a ritual before bedtime that eases you into a restful state. No electronics or television. Even washing up before bed can become a ritual when it is done with the intention of releasing the day. Do these things for a week, and record how you feel in your journal. This practice will help you integrate these new practices into your daily life.

DAY 32

TEN PRINCIPLES OF HAPPINESS, #1

No one is responsible for your happiness. No one gives you happiness. You are its source.

DAY 33

TEN PRINCIPLES OF HAPPINESS, #2

Happiness does not arise from the events in your life; instead, it is constructed as a response to the events in your life.

DAY 34

TEN PRINCIPLES OF HAPPINESS, #3

You get to choose or not to choose happiness. You can choose to stay stuck in an unpleasant situation, or you can move on; or you can transform your interpretation of what is happening, so that you can accept it and take a stance to create something from whatever has occurred.

— DAY 35 —

TEN PRINCIPLES OF HAPPINESS, #4

There are things that make you feel happy and things that make you feel lousy. It makes sense to do more of the former and less of the latter. Integrating your body, mind, and soul makes these activities more meaningful and potent.

— DAY 36 —

TEN PRINCIPLES OF HAPPINESS, #5

When in doubt, help someone else. When you become too self-involved, you are not happy. Understand that nothing in the world allows you to get in touch with your own happiness more than the act of helping someone else. Service is a road to happiness.

— DAY 37 —

TEN PRINCIPLES OF HAPPINESS, #6

Happiness is not a *big* deal; often it's the little details of life that can make you feel the happiest. Petting your dog, swimming in the ocean, eating a sweet strawberry, listening to music, and having a pillow fight with your family all come to mind. What ordinary life events bring you happiness?

— DAY 38 —

TEN PRINCIPLES OF HAPPINESS, #7

Happiness is something you can choose right now. Why wait for it? You may be used to saying, "I'll wait until the weekend, until next year, until the kids are grown up, until I retire," etc. Why not choose to be happy now?

— DAY 39 —
TEN PRINCIPLES OF HAPPINESS, #8

Happiness has to do with how you make meaning and find purpose. It means that you have to pay attention and honor what matters most to you, even if the rest of the world disagrees with you.

— DAY 40 —
TEN PRINCIPLES OF HAPPINESS, #9

Happiness should never become a crutch. Life is an ebb and flow of experiences. Some days those experiences bring you joy, and some days they are more difficult. Learn something from each experience, and that learning will translate into happiness over the course of your life.

— DAY 41 —
TEN PRINCIPLES OF HAPPINESS, #10

A key aspect of happiness is gratitude. In my travels, I have met people from all walks of life and from different cultures. Regardless of the state of their situation, the happiest people are also the ones most filled with gratitude. Be grateful and be happy.

— DAY 42 —
BE CAREFUL WHAT STORIES YOU CREATE

In the absence of information, people create stories and live them as if they were true. Oftentimes the stories we create about each other are far from the truth and based on assumptions we make unconsciously. Question your assumptions and beliefs in order to embrace a larger perspective on life.

DAY 43

CREATE MEANING

Renowned mythologist Joseph Campbell said that we all seek meaning. I see this in my daily conversations with people. Where do you go to seek meaning? How would you recognize it if you "found" it? Meaning is spoken of in terms of being lost or found, as if it were an object outside you. But if it is outside you, if it is something to be found, then what happens when you cannot find it out there? Does that make your life meaningless? And who decides whether your life or my life has meaning? Ultimately, meaning comes from having a deep sense of your essential self. Know yourself, and the rest will fall into place.

DAY 44

FIND THE TREASURE IN YOUR PAST

Have you taken the time to understand yourself well enough to create your meaning, and then to live it? Don't look for it as if it were lost out there. It is not out there—it is within you, created by you.

You and only you decide. Discover it now. Begin by making a list of your fondest memories, starting in your childhood. After you record these memories, notice what they have in common. Are the same people or places present in many of your memories? Perhaps your memories evoke a specific feeling or emotion; what makes you smile about these memories? Take on this assignment as a time-traveling adventure in which you seek out the treasure in your past. By noting what these pleasant memories have in common, you will begin to reconnect with what matters most to you.

— DAY 45 —
TAKE A STAND

The first step in moving toward your essential nature is to decide to do so—to make a declaration in every cell of your body to listen to the song in your soul and to act upon it. Decide. Take a stand. I promise you, the universe will begin to fling doors open when you make this kind of profound declaration.

— DAY 46 —
GO FOR THE GULP!

If you feel safe, you're not living up to your fullest potential. What makes you go "gulp"? Therein lies a clue to what is next for you. Go for that thing!

— DAY 47 —
CONSIDER THE POSSIBILITIES

When you are struggling, either feeling as if your life is out of control or feeling off-balance, consider the following questions, slowly and thoughtfully: What if life were perfect just the way it is right now, without any need to change anything? How would you be living your life? Really, imagine that everything in your life is just right. Don't resist what is. Don't try to change it. If it were perfect just the way it is, what would be possible? What would you be able to do or have?

— DAY 48 —
FIND THE CLUES

Today, ask yourself, "What has helped shape who I am?" Exploring this question will provide clues to the influences that have created your belief systems and worldview.

— DAY 49 —
BECOME A DIFFERENT KIND OF WARRIOR

When you struggle and resist what is, you miss whatever possibilities may exist in the space between what is and what you want to be. It is in this space that you choose suffering or ease. The more you resist, the more you suffer. Sometimes there is more power in the surrender than in the fight. The true warrior must embrace what is in order to be ready for future victories. The paradox may be that to win, sometimes you must surrender.

— DAY 50 —
TELL THE TRUTH

Your greatest fear shows where you are not telling the truth to yourself. What are you most afraid of? Hidden in the shadow is a key to blossoming into a new, more authentic life.

— DAY 51 —
SIMPLIFY

Do you feel as if you are spinning out of control with all that you do and have? Like planets without the sun, you have nothing to ground you if you don't know yourself. Focus on what is essential in your life so you can better manage the roles and responsibilities that come with being you. Eliminate what is no longer useful, whether it means cleaning out your closet of clothes you no longer wear or removing friends from your Facebook page. You will feel lighter afterward.

— DAY 52 —

TRUST THAT LITTLE VOICE

The wise self is that little whisper that you hear distinctly when you don't censor. It is the voice that gives you the very first answer to a profound question. It does not intellectualize or rationalize. It tells you exactly the way things are for you, whether you want to hear it or not. Fear will tell you to doubt the whisper, but be courageous, trust yourself, and follow your own path.

— DAY 53 —

MANAGE YOUR TRANSITIONS

Your life evolves, work changes, relationships wane and grow. Catalysts such as birth, death, marriage, and divorce can move you out of your trance and awaken profound questions in you. By knowing your true nature, you will better manage the transitions in your life. Change is inevitable. Step into the flow of your life, and let your heart lead you to more joy and fulfillment.

DAY 54
BEGIN NOW

In trying times, you may choose the path of least resistance. The world is busy telling you how you cannot and should not want what you want. You decide that the time is not yet right—when you have more money, when the kids are grown, later, later—but too many times, later never arrives. Ask yourself, "If not now, when?" Begin today to work for what you truly want in your life.

DAY 55
A BLUEPRINT FOR LIFE, STEP 1

Stay focused. Do something each day, regardless of how small, to keep your actions moving toward the realization of your dreams or the vision of your business.

— DAY 56 —

A BLUEPRINT FOR LIFE, STEP 2

Get support. Choose to surround yourself with positive people who will act as sounding boards and cheerleaders. This is especially helpful when you are losing momentum or are confronted with obstacles.

— DAY 57 —

A BLUEPRINT FOR LIFE, STEP 3

I am a firm believer in creating a blueprint for what you want, whether that means writing it down, drawing a picture, or having your own personal theme song. Choose something tangible that you can experience or touch each day to remind you of what matters to you. What is that for you? Breathe life into it.

— DAY 58 —

A BLUEPRINT FOR LIFE, STEP 4

Set appropriate goals. When you set your goals according to what holds the most meaning for you, then you move forward with greater ease. Don't set goals based on what you think you should do; instead, keep the vision in mind and ask yourself what about that goal will move you closer to the realization of your vision. Then take action.

— DAY 59 —

A BLUEPRINT FOR LIFE, STEP 5

Allow yourself victories. Don't set your goals or standards so high that you cannot meet them. That will set you up for failure—set yourself up for success instead. Benchmark goals so you can anticipate the feeling of accomplishment that comes from achieving them, and so that you are not so overwhelmed that you take no action at all.

— DAY 60 —
A BLUEPRINT FOR LIFE, STEP 6

Remove energy drains. Take a good look at what drains you. If you are merely tolerating someone or something, remove it from your life or find a solution to dealing with it. This will free up your time and energy and open up a more positive outlook for you.

— DAY 61 —
A BLUEPRINT FOR LIFE, STEP 7

Don't beat yourself up. If things don't go according to plan, resolve the issue as much as you can, then move on and forward. Don't be the person on a diet who in the middle of it binges on ice cream, feels guilty, and then gives up completely because of that one binge. Keep moving.

— DAY 62 —

A BLUEPRINT FOR LIFE, STEP 8

Honor where you have been. There is much to be said for the wisdom that is born of past experiences. Don't throw that out. Sift through your experiences, and use what you can from the past to create a better future.

— DAY 63 —

A BLUEPRINT FOR LIFE, STEP 9

Change course if you think you are struggling. Things may well be difficult, but life really doesn't have to be a struggle all the time. Difficulty and struggle are not the same. If you really want something, your vision for your desired future will take you through difficult situations in ways that prevent you from feeling as if you are struggling. Struggle has an emotional component that includes hopelessness and a sense of disempowerment. Difficulty is just that—difficult—but without hopelessness and disempowerment attached.

— DAY 64 —

A BLUEPRINT FOR LIFE, STEP 10

Energy follows attention. You move toward what you focus on. Focus on avoiding something, and you will move toward it. Focus on creating a new possibility, and you will move toward that, too.

— DAY 65 —

UNCOVER THE OPPORTUNITIES

When my clients are uncomfortable or stuck in their present situation, I often ask this question: "What is the opportunity here?" This allows you to shift your focus to the possibilities that are inherent in every situation. By doing so, you will find that options you may not have considered become available to you. Big shift!

DAY 66
FACE YOUR SCARY PLACES

How often do you find yourself wishing that things were different—and not only wishing that they were different, but actually behaving as if they were what you want them to be? You may be ignoring the truth of what is because it is painful, inconvenient, uncomfortable, more work, even scary. Does this serve you? Does it make sense to put your energy into the fantasy of what you wish could be, instead of addressing what is right in front of you? Would you struggle less if you were accepting what is, rather than operating based on what you wish it were? Today, identify one thing in your life that you are ignoring. Write in your journal what is true and real about that, not about what you would like that thing to be. Then choose one action that you will take, based on that reality, that could open up new possibilities for you.

— DAY 67 —

PAY ATTENTION TO BREAKDOWNS

For every breakdown, an equally powerful break-through is available. You may be taking the path of least resistance until one day everything shatters unexpectedly. What if that breakdown is really the doorway to your bliss? Be present with your breakdowns, learn from them, and notice what possibilities may open on the other side.

— DAY 68 —

MAKE A DIFFERENCE

Do you believe that you can make a difference? Who are you, and what power do you have to impact another individual? Can your existence really make a difference for anyone? At some point in your life, you may begin to recognize a need to have an impact on someone or something. At that point, you may have accomplished much in the way of your material life, yet you may still experience an uncomfortable void or sense of emptiness. Explore what you can contribute in your own community. You don't have to cure world hunger to make a difference.

— DAY 69 —
PRACTICE KINDNESS

Today, focus on the practice of kindness. As you go through your day, how many interactions can you infuse with kindness through your words or actions? At the end of the day, record these inter-actions in your journal and notice how they made both the giver (you) and the receiver feel, and what you learned from them.

— DAY 70 —
PRACTICE GENEROSITY

Today, focus on generosity. As you go about your day, actively seek out ways to express generosity. Don't limit yourself to thinking that generosity has to do with money. Spend a few extra minutes with someone who could use your help. Do something special for someone for no special reason. Donate some time today to a cause you care about. Record your interactions and your observations in your journal.

— DAY 71 —
EXPRESS GRATITUDE

Today, ask yourself, "What's going well right now that I appreciate and want to reinforce?" Incorporate more of these elements into your daily life.

— DAY 72 —
ENGAGE YOUR SHADOW

Notice how easy it is to rejoice in your good fortune when things are going well. It's easy to be kind and generous when you think all is right with your world, but what happens when you experience a setback? How far do you reach into a mindset of scarcity when you lose something? How much doubt enters your mind when you are criticized or when circumstances do not conform to what you expected? How frightened do you get when your safety net is abruptly removed and your complacency is challenged? Answer these questions honestly, and shed light on the shadow places that keep you from being fully present to your life. Write the answers to these questions in your journal. Then add a change of attitude, thinking, or behavior that can counter the dive into fear. Shedding light on those places in us that we keep hidden allows us to free ourselves from fear so that we can continue to live from a loving source. Practice meeting fear with courage and with these new attitudes, thoughts, and behaviors.

— DAY 73 —

MOVE FROM DARKNESS TO LIGHT WITH GRATITUDE

It may become increasingly difficult for you to value what you have when you feel as if your lifestyle or your beliefs have been compromised. Yet it is during the dark moments that it becomes most essential to "see" the light in your life. The stars that can appear in only the darkest skies are the ones that brighten it at midnight. Your experience of this darkest night sky is what will allow you to see twinkling lights. Challenge yourself to look through the eyes of gratitude by writing down one thing each day that you are grateful for. These notes will help you maintain perspective and sustain you in your darkest moments.

— DAY 74 —

DEEPEN YOUR CONNECTION TO OTHERS

There are times that open you to being vulnerable; yet consider that, in being vulnerable, you may also receive unexpected compassion and generosity and love. Vulnerability opens the way to deeper connections with others. Today, if you are feeling a bit lost, take the step of vulnerability and call a valued friend to whom you can open up. This act of reaching out will deepen your friendship and build even more trust between you.

— DAY 75 —

ACKNOWLEDGE WHAT MATTERS MOST

What matters to you? Is it your family, your friends, your skills and abilities, your grace and courage? Be grateful when you see this clearly. Be grateful for the closeness this knowledge brings to your relationships. Today, be thankful for the gift that you are. Surround yourself with people of integrity and people who share your values. Be thankful for your health. Be thankful for love in your life. Be thankful that you can use your body to dance and sing.

— DAY 76 —

FLOW WITH YOUR ESSENTIAL NATURE

Today, ask yourself, "How can I create a life that is in flow with my essential nature? What would that look like? How can I be in alignment with my truest self, rather than creating a life that resists what I am essentially?" Write your thoughts in your journal, and use them as a compass for designing a life of joy and peace.

— DAY 77 —

TELL SOMEONE YOU VALUE HIM OR HER

Think about what friendship really means to you— because true friendship is a precious gift that needs care and nurturing and support. True friendship, much like love, is an engagement of the soul. Whom in your life do you value as a true friend? What is it about that person that is special to you? What are you doing to nurture that friendship? When was the last time you told that person what he or she means to you, despite time, distance, and all that busyness in your life? Share that today.

— DAY 78 —
THREE SHIFTS: SHIFT YOUR PERSPECTIVE

When you want to create something new, you will go through three primary shifts, each one building upon the other. First comes a shift in perspective. You may be holding assumptions or simply not seeing something as possible or available, and thus making excuses for why you cannot possibly have or do something. The shift in perspective happens when your belief in the possibility of something becomes as essential and real as breathing. You begin to actually feel it in your body, mind, and emotions. It becomes a priority for you to attain the quality of life you desire. This moves from being something you have to do as a chore to being something integral to feeling fully alive. You no longer engage in excuses about how difficult it is to do or what might keep you from doing it—you just do it.

– DAY 79 –

THREE SHIFTS: SHIFT YOUR BEHAVIOR

A new perspective makes change begin to happen. What follows is the second shift: behavior. You begin to behave as if you are the person you aspire to be. The shift in perspective also allows you to create a new blueprint. You begin to live within this blueprint of new behaviors and actions. If you want to be a writer, you start incorporating elements of a writing life. If you want to run a marathon, you start training. This does two things: it creates momentum by building upon your first shift in perspective, and it begins to re-create your reality around the goal or vision. It is real and accessible because you are doing it. And all the things that you said would hold you back disappear in the face of this new reality, as you begin to organize your thoughts, behaviors, and actions around it.

— DAY 80 —

THREE SHIFTS: SHIFT YOUR LANGUAGE

Once your perspective has changed and you are taking different actions, you begin to notice the third shift: language. Your language begins to affirm your new perspective in both subtle and overt ways. In manifesting a new shift through language distinctions, you clarify your choices. You stop apologizing for putting your needs first or for making decisions and choices that support your new life. Your language moves from being tentative to being affirmative. Your language becomes more positive and optimistic. It sustains you even during the times when you inevitably meet with obstacles and difficulties. It cements your resolve in a tangible manner.

DAY 81

RECOGNIZE THAT ENERGY FOLLOWS ATTENTION

We create what we focus on. Energy follows attention! Where are you putting your attention? Every moment in your day is energy directed at something. The more attention you give to something or someone, the more energy flows that way. Be aware of how you manage your attention, to ensure that you use your energy to serve your well-being.

DAY 82

SEEK HARMONY, NOT BALANCE

Balance is a concept constructed as an ideal in theory but as a self-defeating goal in reality. Seeking balance is disempowering, because life is too complex and dynamic to maintain balance. You are defeated before you begin. This is especially true for women, who are culturally set up to fail by a society that demands perfect mothers, wives, executives, soccer moms, business owners, and human beings—all at once. Take a holistic and integral perspective, and look at your life as one entity with multiple elements. Assess how all these elements of your life can coexist to support your well-being. Create harmony among all the elements, understanding that there will be occasions that will upset that harmony. Looking at your life holistically can prevent those events that can often push people into breakdowns that last much longer than necessary.

DAY 83

CHOOSE YOUR WELL-BEING

What do you have instead of balance? You have choice. You can make choices that will affect you either positively or negatively. Where are you choosing *for* yourself, and where are you choosing *against* yourself? Note the answers to these questions in your journal, and start making different choices.

DAY 84

SHIFT YOUR ATTENTION INTENTIONALLY

There are times when you may be required to meet deadlines or to do more than normal to meet someone else's needs. You may have set a career goal for yourself that requires more time and dedication. Perhaps your desire to own or grow a successful company means putting other parts of yourself on hold. You choose. You shift the weight from one area of your life to the other. When you maintain a heightened awareness of what is occurring in your life, you are able to intentionally shift your attention between the elements of your life to maintain harmony and well-being.

DAY 85

CHOOSE YOUR BEST LIFE

You control many of the options placed on the scale of life, how long they remain there, and at what point they are removed. Although at any given moment you may not be in harmony, over the course of time, your conscious choices can enable you to shift your attention and energy as needed. You will cease to tolerate what doesn't serve you and will develop a greater acceptance of those things that support your best life.

— DAY 86 —
CREATE BOUNDARIES TO STAY HAPPY AND WELL

Set boundaries around what you will or will not add to your side of the scale. Determine those boundaries based on what you value. At any point, you may need to adjust your immediate requirements, with the intention of bringing yourself back into balance.

— DAY 87 —
CREATE A POSSIBLE FUTURE

Today, ask yourself, "What would it be like if 'it' were even better?" What is "it" for you? Is it your work, your relationships, your health, or something else? Write in your journal what you will do in the next few days to improve your "it."

— DAY 88 —
MOVE WITH WHAT IS

If you have ever sat by a river or an ocean, you know the sensation of being hypnotized by the ebb and flow of the water. Life is similar. During its ebbs, it seems to stand still, and we can use that time to rest and reflect. When it is flowing, it becomes more dynamic, and these times call for action and change. Honor both the ebb and the flow in your life. Where are you today in that cycle?

– DAY 89 –

THANK YOUR HUMAN IMPERFECTION

As a human, you are built to be imperfect. You—all of us—are flawed. Be thankful for that—knowing that you are flawed keeps you more aware of the person you choose to be, someone whose origin is beyond the imperfection and the stupid behaviors that people sometimes manifest at odd times. This human condition is temporary, and beyond what is obvious and visible is an ineffable quality whose source is an infinite fountain of love. That is your true Self, even when you look back to admit mistakes and missteps. One day you will leave this earth, and your conscious-ness will be your compass for the journey home. Stay on the path, and remember who you truly are.

– DAY 90 –

FIND THE LESSON IN THE RIPPLES

A pebble dropped in a still pond is the most basic example we can use to describe what is called the wave interference process. If you drop a pebble into a pond, it creates an infinitely expanding, circular wave pattern. If you drop two pebbles into a pond, the waves' crests eventually meet. The intersecting points of the waves' crests are called the points of interference. The interference of two or more waves will carry all of the information about all of the waves. We could say that we are both the pebble and the wave at the same time. What is intersecting in your life in ways that contribute to your success? Where are the synchronicities playing out, and what are they pointing to? Take a moment to reflect on these questions and see what patterns are emerging in your life.

— DAY 91 —
SEE YOURSELF AS CONNECTED TO HUMANITY

Our world is undergoing trying times. Many individuals and systems are experiencing break-down—and breakthrough. How do you relate your own experience to the larger experience of the human race? How do you relate the experience of the human race to your own experience? Can you see yourself as the pebble in the pond while seeing yourself as the pond itself? Can you be a whole, unique, and separate person while remaining integrated and connected with the larger whole of humanity? What does this inquiry make possible for you? When you consider these questions, stay away from polarizations and dualities. By looking at yourself as integrated with humanity, you will experience a sense of expansion and limitlessness that generates courageous action.

DAY 92
ASK RADICAL QUESTIONS

Like koans, difficult questions require quiet reflection as well as an open mind, heart, and imagination. You may gain a different perspective on your situation. You may find you are not as alone as you believed you were. You may find kinship with those you never even meet. Much is possible from reflecting on radical questions; one radical question is worth a thousand uninspired answers. Write down three radical questions you should be asking yourself right now. Spend some reflective time answering these questions in your journal so you can see new ways of being and acting in the world.

— DAY 93 —

UNCOVER THE OUTSIDE INFLUENCES IN YOUR LIFE

Do you feel as if you are at the mercy of the events in your life? Do you sense that you are not living on purpose but merely following the path of least resistance? Are you the person who takes a job because someone told you it was available and the money was good? Or do you remain in an unfulfilling marriage because it seems like a comfortable habit, never mind that you and your spouse no longer speak or share dreams? Are you the young person who goes to medical school to become a doctor because your father or mother is a doctor? There is no real choosing here. Events or outside influences direct the course of your life, bouncing you from job to job, place to place, and relationship to relationship. In your journal, write down all the ways in which you are living according to outside influences, or what I call "living at cause." Be honest with yourself.

— DAY 94 —
LIVE INTENTIONALLY TODAY

What would it be like to make intentional decisions and choices and to design your life or work with purpose around those things that really matter to you now? This is what I call "living at choice." It means you experience your life with a higher level of awareness that allows you to design your existence in alignment with your essential nature. Where in your life do you need to be more intentional about your choices and decisions? What is one thing you can change to create deeper alignment with your essential nature? Make that change, starting today.

— DAY 95 —
CHOOSE YOUR BOSS

Can you imagine interviewing for a job that you knew met your personal criteria, a job at which you knew you could excel, for an organization to which you could contribute and where you would be acknowledged and rewarded? How much more positive would this experience be for you than your current job is? Would you feel more powerful in this interview knowing that the outcome is as much your choice as it is your prospective employer's. Choose with intention and purpose. The decision is the right one if you make it in alignment with your essential nature.

— DAY 96 —
PAY ATTENTION TO LIFE

Life will always send you lessons to learn, and if you pay attention, you will become more educated. As Rumi says, welcome all of these lessons—"meet them at the door laughing and invite them in." Do not sleepwalk through your life. Be alive and awake! As with a juicy strawberry, let each bite be new; let the juice run down your chin; lick your sticky fingers to capture each drop. Savor all of it.

— DAY 97 —
FIVE COPOUTS, #1: HABITS

There are five things that keep you from getting what you want out of life. I call these the five copouts. The first, habits, are behaviors we have integrated into a routine so much so that we don't realize we do them. We are conditioned to respond over and over again in a particular way, so our responses become thoughtless. What are your habits, and how do they influence your outcomes? Today, concentrate on one or two habits to change and start enacting those changes.

DAY 98

FIVE COPOUTS, #2: FEAR

The "what if" fear, the "but" fear, the "I am not enough" fear, the "what will I lose" fear, the "I might actually get what I want" fear, the "will I be a whole person" fear, the "what will they think" fear, and on and on. . . . Which fear has you? Once you discover that fear, create a new, courageous response.

DAY 99

FIVE COPOUTS, #3: UNAVOIDABLE CIRCUMSTANCES

An example: you have a health issue that requires attention. Within these circumstances, what can you do to eventually reach your aspirations? You can choose to work with the circumstances, or you can remain a victim and fill your life with resentment. How will you choose within your circumstances? Instead of avoiding circumstances, step in and engage them from a place of grounding and courage.

DAY 100
FIVE COPOUTS, #4:
IT'S NOT MY FAULT

Whose fault would it be, if not yours? Does there have to be someone or something to blame? What role do you play in this dynamic that keeps you from your best life? Eventually, you will see that you actually do play a role in every interaction in your life. Where do you need to hold yourself accountable? Once you see that you are part of the dynamic, you can begin to choose on purpose and to take responsibility for your outcomes.

DAY 101
FIVE COPOUTS, #5:
SILENT BELIEFS

These are things you believe about yourself that usually start with "I am," "I am not," "I can't," "I couldn't," and the like. Some examples I have heard are: "I can't do X; I am not smart enough, thin enough, good enough." These beliefs may have been handed down to you, or you may have developed them because of a past event. Either way, they are now so ingrained in you that you can't see that they drive your behaviors and your inaction. What are your silent beliefs? Make a list of those beliefs that have been hiding in the background and keeping you from achieving your dreams, and change them to positive language: "I can," "I am," and so on.

DAY 102

TAKE THE MIND TO THE HEART

When we think love, God is a thought. When we feel love, God is alive in us. Today, stay connected to your feelings and experience this aliveness.

— DAY 103 —
EXPLORE COMMITMENT

The word "commitment" denotes more than a promise to do or not to do something. Making a commitment requires a high level of emotional investment and passion. Without that passionate element, the action or cause may become more of an obligation than a vision that draws you powerfully forward. That passion is also what enables you to move through the inevitable obstacles you encounter in manifesting your dream or vision. For the next few days, we will consider different aspects of commitment that can help guide you in your life. Each day will hold an aspect for reflection.

— DAY 104 —
COMMITMENT: SERVICE

You connect to others through your commitments. When you commit to being in service to others, you connect to your mutual humanity and to enhancing the quality of your life and others' lives.

— DAY 105 —

COMMITMENT: ENVIRONMENT

When you commit to the environment, you are making a deep connection to nature and to living in that connection as a supporting element in the web of life.

— DAY 106 —

COMMITMENT: EDUCATION

When you commit to education, you connect to children and adult learners and teachers, and as such you connect to yourself as teacher or student. When you commit to human rights, you demand for yourself the respect that you seek to ensure for others.

— DAY 107 —
COMMITMENT: CONTRACTS

Commitment supersedes contracts, legal agreements, and other constructs meant to enforce promises. Commitment cannot be regulated. True commitment arises from within, and the contract is merely the outward manifestation of what is true for you internally. True commitment is deeper than contracts. It has more to do with who you are than with what you do.

— DAY 108 —
COMMITMENT: HEART

What you commit to reflects who you are at your deepest level. Being deeply committed to someone or something reflects what really matters to you. It is action driven from your essential self that propels you in a particular direction. It is the heart speaking aloud.

DAY 109
COMMITMENT: COURAGE

Commitment can be frightening. It often asks more of you than you may believe you are capable of. Yet, intuitively, you enter uncharted territory, knowing that in making a commitment, you can begin to realize your dreams. Amazingly, the universe moves in mysterious ways to bring you what you need in order to engage in your new adventure.

DAY 110
COMMITMENT: MOVING ON

There is another side of commitment. What happens when you have fulfilled your commitment and it is time to move on? Or when what you were committed to has ceased to hold the passion and emotional investment for you and may be in the way of your own further development? What is the cost of commitments that are overextended? How do you move on honorably? Where are you experiencing these questions in your life? Identify some place where the commitment needs to come to a clean end, then choose to take action to move on with integrity and clarity.

DAY 111
COMMITMENT: RELATIONSHIPS

When things in your life change, or when you grow apart in a relationship because the passion behind your commitment is no longer present and cannot be resurrected, explore your next steps. I am often asked about how to make this transition. Inherent in the question is the rest of the question: How do I make this transition without hurting anyone? I do not know if these transitions can be made without hurting anyone. The question is less about moving away from a previous commitment and more about how to move toward a new commitment that reflects your evolutionary process. When the dynamics of connections are changed so that expectations are not being met, someone may feel abandoned or hurt. Thus, speaking with honesty, compassion, and integrity is part of making these transitions.

— DAY 112 —
COMMITMENT: HONESTY

Are you being honest about your change in commitment? Do you believe you are leaving this relationship with integrity? Consider one relationship in your life that no longer serves you or the other person and which might even be harmful. Use your journal to write down how you can change that relationship so that it serves both of you.

— DAY 113 —
COMMITMENT: FUNDAMENTALS

Are you putting into place or keeping in place fundamental commitments? Review key commitments, such as care of your children or the referral of a client to another professional. Determine how you can help others to adjust by communicating or by putting other structures in place.

— DAY 114 —
COMMITMENT: ALIGNMENT

Does your new commitment align with your essential nature, your potential, and the values you hold? Instead of thinking of what you will leave behind, focus on what you are choosing for alignment.

— DAY 115 —
COMMITMENT: DISCOMFORT

Are you open to listening to the pain or discomfort of those you leave behind (without needing to "solve" anything)? They may want or need to be heard, even if you can't solve their problem.

— DAY 116 —
ENTER THE SILENCE

There in the place of no words will you discover yourself. Commit to a day of silence and observe what arises. Be gentle with yourself.

— DAY 117 —
CLAIM YOUR BIRTHRIGHT

You are not born fearful. You inherit fear from others. You learn to fear through the messages you receive. Embracing what is possible with wonderment is your birthright. Claim it every day.

— DAY 118 —
BECOME AN ARTIST

What is the picture of your life that you keep recreating? Is that really what you want? Take time today to create a new picture that is the highest expression of your authentic nature.

– DAY 119 –
DO ONE THING

What healthy and positive move will you make for yourself today? Do one thing to feed your spirit, body, mind, and soul.

– DAY 120 –
MOVE CLOSE TO TRUTH

With every step you take in your personal development, you move closer to one thing and further away from something else. You needn't judge this. It is as natural as the changing of the seasons. You have your own seasons and cycles. And with those seasonal changes come new commitments and the dissolution of others. Be intentional about what is important, and you will find that you will know when it is time to move on.

— DAY 121 —
ELEVEN QUESTIONS THAT CAN CHANGE YOUR LIFE

For the next eleven days, I will ask you one question daily, a kind of koan, that could change your life. These are purposely vague so that whatever wants to emerge has the space to do so. Each day, take a moment to reflect on the question and jot down any thoughts or feelings in your journal. This is a reflective exercise and will not require much activity. Allow the questions to work through you. Question #1 is: Why does "it" matter?

— DAY 122 —
QUESTION #2

If this is the end, what is the beginning?

DAY 123
QUESTION #3

If I could do anything in my life, what would I do?

DAY 124
QUESTION #4

What makes my heart sing?

DAY 125
QUESTION #5

If I focused my life around what truly matters, what would I focus on creating?

— DAY 126 —
QUESTION #6

What is at the center of my universe?

— DAY 127 —
QUESTION #7

Who are the most important people in my life, and have I told them what they mean to me?

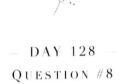

— DAY 128 —
QUESTION #8

If I were bold enough, what would I do that I have not yet done?

— DAY 129 —
QUESTION #9

If I could change one thing about my life in the next thirty days, what would it be?

— DAY 130 —
QUESTION #10

What if the greatest challenge I am facing right now is actually the doorway to my bliss?

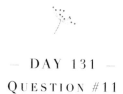

— DAY 131 —
QUESTION #11

What will it take for me to design my life around what truly matters?

— DAY 132 —
CHOOSE LOVE

When faced with a conflict with someone you care for, you have two choices: you can take a defensive stance and raise walls to protect yourself, or you can choose a loving stance, connecting to the other person with your heart and feelings, based on genuine care for the other and for the relationship. Next time you feel the urge to defend, practice choosing love instead, and notice what becomes possible.

— DAY 133 —
START A NEW ADVENTURE

There is no adventure in certainty. Think of your life as a grand adventure! What are the things you would love to do that would be the highest expression of your joy and meaning? Make a list today of the adventures you want to complete in your life.

— DAY 134 —

CREATE A NEW FUTURE STORY

My job is to listen for my clients' stories. It is a privilege to witness another person's story. It is drama, comedy, mystery, and more all tied up in this one human being. What part do you believe so much that it defines you in limiting ways? Begin using the words "Up until now . . ." to speak of your past.

One of my clients claims that she has never been a social person and that networking has always been difficult. Yet as an entrepreneur, she recognizes the need to network to build her visibility. I challenge her to use the words "Up until now, I have not been comfortable networking." And I add, "From this point forward . . . ," and together we begin to write a new story for her—in her case, "From this point forward, I will have one-on-one conversations with people whom I find interesting or with whom I have something in common." She tells me, "Well, I can do that!" And she begins to gradually ease into her new, more expansive story.

— DAY 135 —
WRITE YOURSELF A LETTER

If you could write a letter to your younger self, what would you say to her? What advice would you give her? Today, pause and write a letter to that younger person, sharing the wisdom of your experience.

— DAY 136 —
CHOOSE YOUR STORY

You can choose your story! Which story would you prefer: a story of limitations and defeat, or an empowering story, a bold adventure story, a story of victory? You are the only one writing it!

DAY 137
FOCUS ON THE POSITIVE

What story will you tell me when you sit with me? Will I hear you tell me a story about hurt and disappointment or betrayal of trust? Will I hear self-blame between the lines? Will your body betray your words as you shrink into the soft leather chair in the soft light of my office? Stories remain with us long after the initial event occurs. Some of these stories are alive in a person's mind, body, and spirit, and you can hear that in the tone of voice, or see it in the body. The story becomes a heavy burden on the individual telling the story. If you choose consciously which stories bear repeating and reinforcing and which stories are only one element of your whole experience, you will avoid over-shadowing other elements of your future.

DAY 138
HEAL THE WOUNDS OF YOUR STORY

What is the story you are telling yourself over and over again? What is the story that has you? How does it feel in your body when you tell the story? How does it feel in your heart when you tell the story? What might be an alternative to this story? What do you need to do to heal from the story you tell? How can you gently release the story? And what is the new story you want to create and live? What do you still carry that is best left in the past? Isn't it time to put down your burden? Write a new story, one that is healing and self-affirming. Your past need not dictate your future. There are still many, many stories to write!

— DAY 139 —
LOOK IN THE MIRROR

When you get up in the morning, you can choose to have a positive outlook or a negative outlook. You may not think about this as you are brushing your teeth, but you can choose to begin your day one way or the other. It is not so much about what is happening *around* you as about what is happening *within* you that makes a difference in how your day progresses.

– DAY 140 –
HOLD THE KEY

You hold the key to the wisdom of the universe.
You have only to look into your heart to unlock all
secrets.

– DAY 141 –
TAKE THE FIRST STEP

What is on your mind today? What is there to be
grateful for in this situation? Today, decide what
you want to influence or change, and take one step
toward doing that.

– DAY 142 –
UNDERSTAND YOUR CHOICES

At any given moment, you may choose one thing
over another to achieve a goal or outcome. You may
not have set up your life's framework to support
choosing in alignment with your values. These are

the times when you can feel disempowered. The truth is not that there is no choice, but that you may not like the consequences associated with any of the choices available to you.

— DAY 143 —
MASTER YOUR DESTINY

What needs to be present in order for you to really live your life as a choice? There are key elements that must be present for you to be master of your destiny in a world where you may have very little actual control. During the next couple of days, you will learn what those elements are.

— DAY 144 —
LIFE AS CHOICE:
DEFINE WHAT MATTERS MOST TO YOU

For the next few days, we will look at your life as a choice. Without knowing what is really important to you, you will not be able to make choices that are aligned with the way you envision your life, since good choices cannot be made in a vacuum. Assess your options against a standard of measurement called *personal vision*—a picture of what your ideal life will be.

— DAY 145 —
LIFE AS CHOICE:
CREATE A STRUCTURE

Create a structure that supports getting what you need and want with minimal struggle and fear. You are apt to make choices driven by fear, instead of making choices directed by creativity and authenticity, if you haven't planned to have what you want in your life. As an example, when you are faced with a job evaluation, you can entertain thoughts such as *I should be grateful to have a job or to get any raise at all*, when in reality you have performed above your employer's standards and deserve to ask for and receive a raise or some other compensation. But you don't negotiate, for fear that you may be left with less or nothing. Consider some options—you can remain in a job that drains you or that you resent, adapt to the present job, or move to another job that is meaningful and rewarding. At some point, the balance will shift. Why wait until you are in so much pain that you cannot plan to be successful?

— DAY 146 —
LIFE AS CHOICE:
PLAN FOR GOOD STUFF

Anticipate those things that matter to you, and plan to have them in your life. If you really want to retire at forty, then create a plan, a life framework, that supports that goal. If you know you want to have children and also want to continue on your career path, identify what actions you need to take now to bring this about later. Not creating a plan is like not making a decision—a non-plan, like a non-decision, is a decision in itself, a decision of non-choice.

DAY 147
LIFE AS CHOICE:
WANT WHAT YOU HAVE

You can't have it all, all the time. Life is just not set up that way. The concept of having it all is a setup for exhaustion and sabotages you. The key isn't having what you want; it's wanting what you have. There is peace in accepting and engaging from exactly where you are. It is the only way to know what steps may be next on your journey.

DAY 148
LIFE AS CHOICE:
DIFFERENTIATE BETWEEN CHOICE
AND DECISION

Understand the distinction between choice and decision. A decision has to do with two options; a choice includes multiple options. When you are faced with a decision, ask yourself if there are other options you might not have considered. For example, you like your job and the company, but you don't like the work. The decision may limit you to staying or leaving. Staying and moving to another department, adjusting your job responsibilities, and asking for flexible hours are all options that you might explore before you resort to either/or decisions. But here again, you must know what matters most to you in order to negotiate for, ask for, and plan for a meaningful assignment.

— DAY 149 —
LIFE AS CHOICE:
ALIGN YOUR CHOICES WITH
YOUR GOALS

You are not responsible for how others respond to your choices. Everyone has an opinion about how you choose, but you are not responsible for their point of view or their response to your choices. Others may be affected, but your purpose is not to change others; it's to align your choices with how you want your life to be. There is only one way to fail, and that is to try to please everyone.

— DAY 150 —

LIFE AS CHOICE:
BECOME INCLUSIVE AND HOLISTIC

Add "and" to your vocabulary. The use of the word "and," instead of "or," will point to other options. This is a very simple but effective shift. Practice it today.

— DAY 151 —

LIFE AS CHOICE: BREAK OLD HABITS

Habits and cycles keep us from choice. You have a lifetime of developing habits and getting caught up in negative cycles. When you become self-aware, you notice these habits. Break old, ineffective habits. Determine what you need to do, or undo, to break cycles. If you have been overworking to keep up with projects to the point of exhaustion, is working late hours actually effective and helpful to you or your clients? Do the opposite: get out of work at a reasonable hour, spend time with your family or on things you enjoy, and get rest so you are most effective. Break the workaholic cycle.

— DAY 152 —

LIFE AS CHOICE: CHOOSE DIFFERENTLY THAN YOU HAVE IN THE PAST

Know that your choices, and how you make them, will change. As your life evolves and includes other life events, what matters to you may change, and so will your choices. The key is to be aware that who you are today and what you need today may not be the same as yesterday or tomorrow. Choose for today. There are only a few decisions that impact your whole life. Keep this perspective when you make your choices and decisions. To make it easier, begin by saying, "For now, I will . . ." It is just for now.

— DAY 153 —

LIFE AS CHOICE: EMBRACE REALITY

There can be limited choices. Times of extreme stress—such as a long period of unemployment, a divorce, single parenthood, or a financial catastrophe—will limit your options, and you may find it necessary to make choices based on the fundamental need to survive. Don't judge these survival-based choices against the choices you make when your circumstances are more flexible. If you have been out of work for a long time and have a family to support, you may have to take any job to provide income until times are better. But remember, these times are usually temporary and these decisions are not permanent. Times of stress illustrate the importance of creating a supportive life framework early on to assist you in challenging times.

— DAY 154 —
LIFE AS CHOICE:
USE COURAGE AS A CREATIVE FORCE

Even in times of great stress, even in times when you are feeling powerless, the knowledge that you can still choose how you respond can give you strength and courage. Apply this courage to create strategies in your daily life so you will come to experience life as a choice.

— DAY 155 —
CREATE HARMONY

I often think of Mother Nature and the harmony that is created even out of chaos. I notice weather patterns in nature and the ebb and flow of the tides. Nature's harmony takes into account the whole system, not merely one or two aspects of it. Start looking at your life as a whole system, and notice where you see disharmony or imbalance. Write about this in your journal, and identify ways you can recalibrate to create harmony.

— DAY 156 —
PLAY WITH A KOAN

What does the following statement mean to you: "If you want to go sailing, you don't drop anchor"? Be playful with this koan.

– DAY 157 –
RECALIBRATE AGAIN AND AGAIN

When you affect or influence one area of your life, inevitably other areas will also be affected. For example, if you are hired for a new job, you may have to allow more time for commuting, which means you may have to move your day care from one town to another, which means you may need to allot more money to pay for that day care, and on and on. Remain aware that one change will affect multiple areas of your life.

– DAY 158 –
CREATE SYNERGY IN YOUR LIFE

Balance is a duality. Harmony is integral and whole. You are either in or out of balance. Harmony seeks a synergy of multiple parts of the whole that allows for flexibility, expansion, and contraction—perhaps all at the same time—in order to keep the entity, person, or organization fluid, healthy, and thriving.

Take an inventory of your life, and notice where synergy allows things to flow and where there is resistance. Move toward the flow of your life.

— DAY 159 —
BUILD AWARENESS OF YOUR ENVIRONMENT

Harmony allows for more choices and more areas to balance out, not just two areas. If you consistently think in terms of maintaining harmony, instead of balance, you will have additional reserves of energy, time, money, or resources for those times when you meet with the unexpected, and you will have more options for being successful. Harmony allows for more flexibility as it increases your awareness of your environment.

— DAY 160 —
WEATHER THE STORMS

Consider nature your teacher. Next time there is a storm, watch the natural elements. Notice how all the elements interact and shift in response to the storm. Your life, whether sunny or stormy, is similar, and seeking harmony will help you lead a life with more flow and ease.

— DAY 161 —
ACCEPT THE UNACCEPTABLE

Where in your life are you feeling stress from a situation that is not what you want it to be? What about this is unacceptable? What would happen if you could accept this situation? What possibilities or outcomes might arise from this shift in perspective? There are always things that are truly unacceptable, but if you begin by asking this question, you may find that accepting what is unacceptable is the first real step in transforming your circumstances.

— DAY 162 —
BUILD A CATHEDRAL

Every day you can choose whether you will start your day as a bricklayer or as a builder of cathedrals. Every day you can look in the mirror and choose your own greatness or choose to be the victim of circumstances. Based on that choice, you will experience your day accordingly.

— DAY 163 —
TAKE CARE WITH YOUR INTENTIONS

Intention is the first step in reaching your potential. Your intention focuses you on the correct actions and behaviors that will produce a desired outcome. Your intention will either inspire you or create struggle.

— DAY 164 —
DRIVE WITH INTENTION

Intention is the foundation, and action is the driver that moves your intention into reality. If you intend to be a partner in your firm, then you will behave as one. If you intend to be a caring parent (or son or daughter), you will behave with care and affection. If you intend to hide from life, then you will behave as if your actions do not matter.

— DAY 165 —
BE FULLY ALIVE NOW

Are you still waiting for "someday"? The essence to living life to the fullest is presence and awareness. To be fully alive is to be fully present and conscious, to all of it, without making judgments about good and bad. That way, you can receive all of life with open arms, and when it's time to go, you can leave gracefully with empty hands.

DAY 166

CREATE POSSIBILITIES

Are you busy avoiding problems, or would you prefer to create possibilities? The energy associated with doing one as opposed to the other is vastly different. Which would you prefer? You choose— and you choose each and every day you look in that mirror.

DAY 167

DEVELOP YOUR PERSONAL CRITERIA

Possibilities are not opportunities. They are what is possible. The real question is, "Is this right for me?" If the answer is yes, then you are looking at an opportunity. But what is possible is not always what is optimal or best for you. There is a subtle gap between possibility and opportunity. What tran- scends that gap has to do with your "personal criteria" or your values—what really matters to you.

DAY 168

FOLLOW YOUR CRITERIA

Possibility or opportunity? You will know the answer to this question only when you are crystal clear about what really matters to you. When you can give yourself permission to weigh your possibilities against your personal criteria without judgment, you will discover your true opportunity. It may surprise you when you choose what you really want or need over the strident, judgmental voice of your mind and the well-meaning advice of others. Only you know your personal criteria—whatever they are, stay true to them to enjoy a life of joy and harmony.

DAY 169

ELIMINATE WHAT DOES NOT SERVE YOU

Take the following challenge: eliminate one thing this week that takes up your time and energy and does nothing to align with your truest nature. Did you feel that pang in your stomach—the *oh, no, not that!* feeling? Explore what that pang is telling you, and use your courage to move beyond the feeling into one decisive action today.

DAY 170
CLEAN UP YOUR CALENDAR

At least 40 percent of what is on your calendar is there to make you feel good about yourself. It proves that you are that high achiever, the go-getter, the go-to person at the office or at home. Like cleaning out your closets, clean out your calendar and clean out your life. Remove the nonessentials by consciously assessing the reason you are saying yes to the commitments you make. As you eviscerate your calendar, new blank spaces will light up your screen, inviting you to fill them in again. Resist the urge!

— DAY 171 —
EMBRACE AUTHENTICITY

Today, ask yourself, "What is the gift that is not being expressed in my life or my work?" These gifts can remain hidden when you do not embrace your true nature. Explore the question by standing in your authenticity.

— DAY 172 —
BE PROACTIVE ABOUT YOUR LIFE

Why wait for the worst circumstances to learn what is essential and nonessential? Be proactive, and take some time now to clean out your life. In those blank spaces, you will find quiet and the energy to flow with the life you really desire.

— DAY 173 —

CHOOSE YOUR FRIENDS AND YOUR ACTIVITIES

Consciously begin to choose whom you spend time with and what you spend your time doing. First, keep the essentials: those people and activities that support the way you choose to lead your life. These may include your health, your friends or family, hobbies, or spiritual practice. Notice how these are exactly the things that place last in the race for time. Change the course of your day by placing these first and then assessing what you need or want to include after these. Nonessential activities drain you and often anchor you to a way of life that is void of passion and spirit.

— DAY 174 —

THREE PRACTICES FOR PRODUCTIVITY, #1: DO IT

If it is something you can handle right on the spot, then do it. As the adage goes, don't leave for tomorrow what you can do today. Doing it, however, means consciously leaving time in your day to handle things. It means not packing your schedule so tightly that you cannot handle those things that can easily be managed and taken care of. This frees up not only your time but also the psychic space that having something hanging over you will consume.

— DAY 175 —
THREE PRACTICES FOR PRODUCTIVITY, #2: DUMP IT

Though this is perhaps not very eloquently stated, it is nevertheless a viable strategy. Do you hold on to your e-mails or to-do lists, only to find them, a month later, somehow resolved without any consequence? I believe there must be a pack-rat gene in us somewhere that makes us hold on to so much, when the wisest course of action is to make a decision to release what isn't relevant. In the case of work, if it turns out to be the wrong decision, surely someone, somewhere, will have a copy of it.

— DAY 176 —
THREE PRACTICES FOR PRODUCTIVITY, #3: DELEGATE IT

This is another tough one. It instantly triggers the "what ifs." ("What if someone else doesn't do it right, as well as I do, completely, etc.?" "What if it gets lost in the shuffle?" "What if . . . ?") Delegation is a learned skill, so practicing it is important.

— DAY 177 —
WORK WITH COMPETENT PEOPLE

Choose to work with or hire people who are competent, dedicated, and self-motivated, and you will not have a problem delegating. Consider that delegating is not the same as abdicating. To delegate, make sure you are making your requests clear and specific, and make sure that the person to whom you delegate work has the skills and tools to perform the work and is motivated to do his or her best.

DAY 178
EMPOWER OTHERS

Rather than doing everything yourself, mentor others to surpass their current skills. As you empower others around you to take responsibility, you will free yourself to focus on what matters at work, and those people will feel successful, learn, and grow.

DAY 179
RETURN TO THE THREE "D"S

Repeat the three "D"s to yourself like a mantra: *Do it. Dump it. Delegate it.* When you are suddenly inspired to deal with your inbox or the piles of papers and folders on your desk, ask yourself which "D" is the right one to handle your overwhelming amount of stuff. Get used to asking if you should do it, dump it, or delegate it right now. Keep your outer space organized, and your inner space will feel calm and harmonious as well.

DAY 180
THE FOUR BANK ACCOUNTS: TIME

There are four primary methods of exchange that you can use to get things done. I call these the Four Bank Accounts. Overusing one will cause you to go bankrupt in that area. You will want to stay alert to depositing into each account to keep all of them replenished and available for you to access when you need something.

First, there is time. If you had more time, you could . . . fill in the blank! Time seems to be the most precious commodity these days. You may enjoy cooking and want to spend time entertaining friends. What's another bank account you could use to buy some time?

DAY 181
THE FOUR BANK ACCOUNTS: MONEY

A good example here is paying for housekeeping. If indeed you do not want to withdraw from your time bank account, another option is to pay for services. This literally buys you time to spend otherwise.

— DAY 182 —
THE FOUR BANK ACCOUNTS: RESOURCES

You have resources and your friends have resources that, if pooled and shared, could help you better manage your lives. Maybe your neighbor loves to decorate, and you would like to redecorate your home. Maybe the high school boy or girl next door needs a letter of recommendation in exchange for some office work. Maybe you can borrow some tools for a household project and return them when you are done, thereby saving yourself the cost of buying tools that you would use only occasionally. Bartering and borrowing are age-old exchanges of resources that work particularly well when the participants clearly state their expectations.

— DAY 183 —

THE FOUR BANK ACCOUNTS: ENERGY

Using physical, mental, or emotional energy can be invigorating or draining. How much energy are you willing to commit to accomplishing something? Is that where you would like to place your energy? Some examples of using your energy might be keeping in touch with friends who live far away, or volunteering. As you invest your energy in these relationships or tasks, you may reap fulfilling rewards.

— DAY 184 —

CHANGE THE WAY YOU
GET THINGS DONE

Instead of asking, "How am I going to do this?" ask, "How will this get done?" By asking the last question, you explore more options and can determine which bank account you can use. Don't over-withdraw from one bank account. If you do, soon enough you will be bankrupt in time, money, resources, *and* energy. Whether it's about managing your money well or about managing your time, energy, and resources, use these accounts for investing in a full and happy life that gives you what truly matters to you.

— DAY 185 —
MANAGE YOUR CAREER

Your career is a fundamental element in your life. Your personal life and your career should coexist harmoniously in order for you to feel at ease. Take time periodically to assess your career and check in on your future aspirations. You may find you need to add something or change something else to keep yourself on track. Take some time today to do an assessment of your career. Identify where you are in the flow and where you may need to change things, using the following coping strategies as a guide.

DAY 186

COPING STRATEGIES, WORK AND CAREER, #1: INVEST IN YOURSELF

The idea of company as parent is an anachronism. You are responsible for your career. The sooner you begin to invest in yourself, the more prepared you will be for the uncertainty of the future. You cannot control the economy or the way decisions are made in organizations, but you *can* control your ongoing learning, your résumé, and your marketability, so be proactive about your career.

DAY 187

COPING STRATEGIES, WORK AND CAREER, #2: GET EMOTIONAL

If you have lost your job, deal first with the emotional aspects. You may experience a sense of betrayal. (*How could this have happened, when I was so good at my job?*) You may experience feelings of guilt (*What did I do wrong?*) or of anger, loss, and frustration. First, understand that all of these emotions are normal. Ask for assistance with handling them so that they do not paralyze you or make you ill. Remember, you are not what you do; you are not your job.

DAY 188

COPING STRATEGIES, WORK AND CAREER, #3: LOOK FOR THE OPPORTUNITY

This is particularly difficult if you have recently lost your job and have not addressed the emotions that resulted from that experience. Yet, this may an ideal time for you to assess what you liked and disliked about that job and to look toward choosing your future job with more purpose and a clearer idea of your value and what you need to feel successful. If you are laid off, negotiate a severance package that gives you some financial cushion to pursue the opportunities that best suit you.

— DAY 189 —

COPING STRATEGIES, WORK AND CAREER, #4: DECIDE WHAT MATTERS

If there is one thing you should know, it is that every moment is precious—and tenuous. Don't grasp for what may be available out there. Instead, look for meaningful work and intentionally choose the organizations with which you want to be aligned. Be the driver, not the passenger, in your career.

— DAY 190 —

COPING STRATEGIES, WORK AND CAREER, #5: DON'T DO IT ALONE

Move out into the world of work with confidence. Get assistance from a coach or counselor, and from friends and family. Get professional help in writing a cover letter or résumé. The rules of career management have changed. Read and become knowledgeable about a career or job change. You have less than thirty seconds to get the attention of a prospective employer. Make it count.

— DAY 191 —

COPING STRATEGIES, WORK AND CAREER, #6: MAINTAIN PERSPECTIVE

If you have lost your job, remind yourself that this is not a life-threatening or terminal situation. Although nothing is certain, you can find opportunity by tapping your network of contacts.

— DAY 192 —

COPING STRATEGIES, WORK AND CAREER, #7: SET REASONABLE GOALS FOR YOURSELF

Set appropriate goals for your job search, using your values as the standard of measurement. Work on your job search, but don't forget you have a life outside of that. Maintain your health and well-being by including social, fitness, and other activities that bring you happiness and benefit you. You will exude health and a positive attitude, which are very attractive when it comes to interviews and networking.

— DAY 193 —

COPING STRATEGIES, WORK AND CAREER, #8: DEVELOP YOUR NETWORK

Cultivate your network at all times. The wider the career net you cast, the greater your chances of success will be. Make a list of everyone you might consider a resource in your job search. Contact each one and convey your ideas about the type of position you would like and for which you would be qualified. Then make a direct request for assistance or for a referral to someone else who might bring you closer to your next job. The Internet is a wonderful job search tool, but nothing compensates for face-to-face interactions.

— DAY 194 —

COPING STRATEGIES, WORK AND CAREER, #9: DON'T GET DISCOURAGED

If you are in the midst of a job search, keep in mind that the average hunt may last longer than you expect. Organizations don't hire according to your timetable. Don't assume the worst if you do not hear back from someone.

— DAY 195 —

COPING STRATEGIES, WORK AND CAREER, #10: TAKE A BREAK

If you feel yourself getting frustrated, re-energize yourself. Re-strategize. Get another perspective from an objective person to uncover any gaps you may not be aware of.

— DAY 196 —

COPING STRATEGIES, WORK AND CAREER, #11: CONSIDER FREE AGENCY

Have you considered that maybe you aren't cut out for the corporate, nine-to-five lifestyle? Collaborate with others who may be aligned with your business philosophy and with your talents and skills. Again, your personal relationships and networking skills will play an important role in your success as a free agent. Maybe finding work, as opposed to finding a job, is appropriate for you for a while.

DAY 197

COPING STRATEGIES, WORK AND CAREER, #12: BE PROACTIVE

The nature of career and work is changing dramatically. In Career Thought Leaders' white paper "2013 Global Career Brainstorming Day," the researchers explore the role of social media and personal branding, as well as the needs of the global economy, as they relate to career management. Being proactive about your career is still the best strategy for achieving satisfying work. Validate your work and your competency from the inside out. Keep a success or accomplishments log. Maintain your networking contacts and an updated résumé. Having these in place will keep you ready to move whenever an opportunity presents itself.

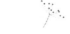

DAY 198

CREATE ACTION

Over the course of a day, we have many conversations. Some of them are relational, where we build friendships and connections with one another.

Others are what I call conversations for action. There are conversations that promote forward motion.

Over the next five days, I'll introduce you to conversations for action; each day offers a specific lesson for you to practice. Today, watch your conversations and identify which are conversations for action and which are other kinds of conversations. That will prepare you for tomorrow.

DAY 199
CONVERSATIONS FOR ACTION: INTENTION

You will reap exactly what you ask for, so, as the saying goes, be careful what you wish for. If your intention is to inform and educate, understand that this is a one-way conversation and that little beyond that will occur. If your conversation has been initiated for selling or marketing purposes—for instance, to close a deal or get clients—then informing will not be enough. How you create the conversation to inform is very different than creating a conversation to get clients. Set the stage early by stating up front what the desired result is and how you and others will recognize the conversation as complete. In cases of negotiation—whether it is with your spouse or with your boss—be clear about what you really want and what you are or are not willing to trade to get that outcome. Today, practice writing down the intentions behind significant conversations you will have today.

— DAY 200 —
CONVERSATIONS FOR ACTION: PERSPECTIVE

A friend of mine, Paul Rezendes, a tracker and photographer in Massachusetts, once told me about a concept he calls "splatter vision." It is the kind of vision that allows him to see the signs on the ground while being aware of a deer standing just yards away. He speaks of the ability to basically see the details as you see the bigger picture. You need splatter vision, too. To have a conversation for action, you must focus on the details of your communication while communicating within the larger context of your goals and your desired action. Today, practice connecting the details of your communication to a larger context and desired action.

— DAY 201 —
CONVERSATIONS FOR ACTION: COMMUNICATION

You communicate with your body, with your words, and with your tone. Notice when your communication is fully congruent with the action you desire. For example, to negotiate from strength, you do not look at the floor and use tentative language. The appropriate use of language and metaphor can be very powerful in your conversations for action. Today, notice where there is incongruence between your words and your tone or body language. It might be helpful to notice this in others first and see how that makes you feel.

— DAY 202 —
CONVERSATIONS FOR ACTION: FOCUS

Your conversations for action must be structured around the result you want to achieve. Each element of such a conversation must align with and support this focus. Engaging in irrelevant conversation will diminish the urgency or the importance of the desired result. Today, when you start an important conversation, begin it by stating your focus or goal, and then use the conversation to support your stance.

— DAY 203 —

CONVERSATIONS FOR ACTION: COMPLETION

Determine at what point the conversation is complete. Do not walk away with unspoken expectations, or without asking the other person if the conversation is complete and receiving a confirmation of the action that is now required. Defining the desired result and the criteria for completion at the start of the conversation will move the conversation forward in a focused manner and will point to the conclusion when it arrives. In your conversations today, begin by stating the reason for your conversation and what your desired outcome is. Before you leave the conversation, ask directly if you and the other person are both in agreement that the conversation is complete. You may find that others will understand your communications better and that you have communicated in a way that allows their ideas to be expressed as well.

— DAY 204 —
IDENTIFY YOUR ASSETS AND LIABILITIES

Your greatest asset is your greatest liability as well. If you are very creative, you may have a tendency toward ideas but not follow through. If you are task-oriented, you may have a tendency to become mired in the details. If you are decisive and assertive, are you incorporating personal and emotional skills to communicate your objectives? You will lean on your strengths so much that at some point, they may become your liabilities. Where do your strengths lie, and at what point do they become a liability to you? Distinguish where this limit is, and practice stopping before that limit and recalibrating so that your strengths move you in a positive direction.

— DAY 205 —
SHIFT THE CONVERSATION

The more conversation you have around what tethers you, the longer you remain in the same place. Shift the conversation to what you want to create, and move toward that. Focus on activities and actions that you know will lead you toward your goals. In the case of work, you may want to join different associations and become active in those. In your personal life, you may want to join a local fitness group to create a healthier lifestyle.

— DAY 206 —
STEP OUT OF YOUR COMFORT ZONE

What ideas do you protect? Where did your assumptions come from? Do you keep repeating the same pattern of thinking and action? Despite its being proven ineffective, you may still cling to your comfort zone and keep repeating the same action or choosing the same belief or approach. Is it better to be comfortable than to be happy? Are you finding answers doing what you have been doing? Is it time to change your thinking? Notice your thoughts— they will illustrate hidden beliefs, assumptions, and limitations you hold.

DAY 207
CHANGE COURSE

What approach do you keep repeating? What outcome do you fear will occur if you start doing things differently? What is really at stake? What could you do that would be radically different? If you are not achieving your goals despite expending energy and effort, review what you keep doing over and over, and make changes to conserve or redirect that energy.

— DAY 208 —
DO SOMETHING RADICAL

Get uncomfortable, do something totally different, and see if you don't reap more than you did before. One shy client of mine decided to join a dinner group. It was out of her comfort zone and so was a radical move for her, but she now has a group of friends who enjoy cooking as much as she does. Another of my clients had never traveled internationally, until she took a trip by herself to Italy, where she met other women traveling and had what she calls the best experience of her life. Do something radical and positive this week.

— DAY 209 —
SYNCHRONICITY HAPPENS

When you change how you are in the world, you may find synchronicity appearing to affirm your new choices. It may appear as a chance meeting or as a possibility that challenges your belief of self. Notice!

— DAY 210 —
EMBRACE COSMIC CHUCKLES

When you are paying attention, you will begin to see what I call "cosmic chuckles," which will cause you to laugh at yourself as you notice that something has shifted. In recognizing this, you can then fully step into this new chapter and own all of who you are becoming. Your powerful self is emerging!

— DAY 211 —
EMPOWER YOURSELF

The world is apt to tell you how you will fail before it tells you how you will succeed. Listen to your own wisdom and empower yourself by remaining true to your essential nature and aligning with that. When the world tells you that you can't, simply reply, "Thank you for sharing your opinion" and continue on your way to joy.

— DAY 212 —
TAKE A RISK

Today, ask yourself, "What is so compelling that I am willing to take a risk for it?" Risk is frightening because you believe that you will experience loss when you change—but what are the risks in staying the same? You may find that the status quo is more frightening than the change you wish to make.

— DAY 213 —
BREATHE

The word "inspiration" comes from the Latin meaning "to breathe." Breath is life. When we breathe deeply, everything in our body and our energetic fields moves. The breath makes more love, more courage, and more faith available to us. Today, breathe deeply and be grateful for life.

— DAY 214 —
TAP YOUR FOUNTAIN OF CREATIVITY

Inspiration suggests both a creative element and imagination. Inspiration can also suggest a spiritual element, something that is born from your essential Self and calls to you to manifest an idea, a dream, or a vision. Inspiration evokes emotions, energizes you, and provokes action. When you are creating, inspiration moves you through the difficult and uncomfortable place of uncertainty and not knowing. It sustains you through doubts and obstacles.

— DAY 215 —
BE AN INSPIRED PERSON

How does your style, presence, or language affect those around you? Are you inspiring them or motivating them? Each force has its own place and value. Be aware which one you are tapping. What would it be like to inspire greater potential in others? When those around you are inspired, their level of commitment to a vision or goal increases. This energy is contagious and can bring about higher levels of productivity and satisfaction in you.

— DAY 216 —

BECOME AN INSPIRED LEADER

What shifts would need to occur for you so that you could inspire others? What role does inspiration play in your life? How do you inspire yourself? Look around you for others who may inspire you, and follow their lead.

— DAY 217 —

INSPIRE SOMEONE ELSE

To inspire someone is powerful. Inspiration does not require an outside force; it flows without struggle and draws you toward something. This is more powerful than motivation, whose progress may depend on outside stimulation or incentive. Once that incentive is removed, are you still motivated? If you are not motivated, check in with yourself for a deeper, more personal meaning, one beyond an outside incentive, that will keep you moving forward for the sake of your own development.

DAY 218
MAKE THE MOST OF YOUR INTERACTIONS

Each time you interact with someone is an opportunity to inspire and be inspired. Pay attention. Stay in touch with your inner world. Be generous, and inspiration will find you.

DAY 219
HAVE FAITH

Today, ask yourself, "How is my life an act of faith?" Start your day with the faith that life will reveal itself to you through tiny miracles if you can open your eyes to them today.

— DAY 220 —
EXPLORE FOCUS

Today and for the next twelve days, you will explore focus and the elements thereof that can help you better manage your life. From my work with many successful CEOs, I have learned that they schedule only about 40 percent of their time and leave the rest available to deal with issues that arise, and to reflect and strategize. Successful leaders operate in the quadrant of important/not urgent. This allows them to have long-range vision on issues that are important but not necessarily urgent. Crisis management exists in the quadrant of important/urgent. Too much time here causes burnout and creates an environment for faulty decision making.

— DAY 221 —
ON FOCUS: IMPORTANT OR URGENT?

How much time do you spend in the important/urgent quadrant? How can you move into the important/not urgent quadrant? Answer: don't overschedule yourself. Keep time in your day both to work strategically on achieving your goals and for quiet reflection. This will allow you to move forward bit by bit and still work tactically during the day. You will retain focus because the time you set aside is consistent and specifically for thinking and reflection. You will notice that actions derived from this time are more targeted, preemptive, and successful.

— DAY 222 —
ON FOCUS: ONE THING AT A TIME

Just as you can be in only one place at one time, you can focus on only one thing at one time. Although we have come to value multitasking, in reality splitting our attention is not useful. Be there in the moment with what is present, deal with it, and then move on to the next task. Trying to be in multiple mental places at the same time doesn't work. Deal with each link in the time chain, moving smoothly from one link to another, until it is complete. This presence will lead you to the inevitable conclusion that by concentrating on what action is needed from moment to moment, you will reach your goal without feeling drained and fatigued.

— DAY 223 —

ON FOCUS: POSITIVE MOVEMENT

There is a difference between something that draws you forward and something that pushes you away. For example, if you are in a career transition, are you approaching it as a way to leave your current job (pushing away), or as a way to create a life and work around what matters most to you (drawing you forward)? Each of these approaches contains a very different energy. You will flow toward the creation of new work, but you will get stuck running away from the current situation. Think in terms of moving toward something, as opposed to moving away from something, and you will be better able to maintain focus.

— DAY 224 —

ON FOCUS: YOUR IDEA FOLDER

Creative people have particular difficulty maintaining focus over the long term. When I ask my most creative clients what gets in the way, they inevitably point to all the ideas that they conceive and the distractions that doing so generates. An effective solution is to create an idea folder where you can capture ideas for a later date. Knowing that these ideas are available for implementation later is likely to appease the creative mind in the short term and provides long-term fodder for new projects.

— DAY 225 —
ON FOCUS: THE MAGNIFYING GLASS

Having focus does not mean excluding other tasks, ideas, or projects. Focus means that *for now* you will concentrate your efforts on one task, idea, or project. Think of a magnifying glass. When the rays of the sun pass through the magnifying glass, they narrow and ignite the paper on the other side. That does not mean that the sunlight around the magnifying glass is extinguished. Such is the same with focus. You still have other things to do, but your energy, time, and resources are concentrated on one thing. Today, choose one thing that you need to complete, and focus on that. Once you complete it, move to the next thing. Be sure to acknowledge your success!

— DAY 226 —

ON FOCUS: A POWERFUL QUESTION

Create an orientation first, and then use a powerful question to help you to decide minute by minute how you will use your time, energy, and resources. For example, "I want to increase sales by $5,000 this month," or "I want to run a marathon next year." That becomes the orientation. The focusing question that you would then ask when confronted with options on how to spend your time might be: "What action or behavior brings me closer to my goal of +$5K or running a marathon next year?" You orient your actions around your desired result. You will make better decisions with greater ease and maintain focus.

— DAY 227 —

ON FOCUS: RELATIONSHIPS

If your goal is to have a committed relationship, this also works. What actions, beliefs, or approaches will bring you closer to meeting someone who is interested in a committed relationship with you?

Answering these questions will help you to clarify the qualities of your ideal partner, and your chances of finding this person will increase.

— DAY 228 —
ON FOCUS: OPTIONS

Having options is a wonderful thing, but in today's culture, we are barraged with too many. Ultimately, the brain can choose from only two options, so reduce yours to this amount and eliminate your analysis paralysis in the process.

— DAY 229 —
ON FOCUS: A KOAN

Which came first, the chicken or the egg? This is a Western koan. The answer is: yes! Ultimately, you end up making it all up anyway, so decide, take action, and move in the direction of your goals and dreams.

— DAY 230 —
ON FOCUS: AWARENESS

How do you choose to spend this one moment? This question is designed to increase your awareness of the intentional choices you make. You may choose to do something you don't really want to do, but you are choosing mindfully and on purpose. Choosing intentionally reduces stress and increases confidence.

— DAY 231 —
ON FOCUS: A MANTRA

Develop a mantra that can help you focus on what you want to achieve. An example for someone who is committing to his wellness is *get strong.* This is a simple, concise, and powerful mantra—the best kind! For someone who is pursuing greater leadership possibilities at work, the mantra could be *I lead through community.* What mantra can you create to evolve yourself? Write it down, place it somewhere you can see it throughout the day, and keep repeating it today. This act will generate positive energy that moves you toward what you want to create.

— DAY 232 —
ON FOCUS: ATTENTION

You may have big plans, but without intention, focus, structure, support, and action, they may well remain just that. Focus starts with quality of attention. When you are paying attention to what is around you, when you place yourself in the role of observer, your quality of attention increases and you are able to maintain your focus on your goals. The higher the quality of your attention, the more focus you will have and the more assured you will be in designing your work and life around what truly matters to you.

— DAY 233 —
NOTICE ABUNDANCE

When you are tired or feeling overwhelmed, it is easy to lose sight of the abundance that is present right in front of you. There is a Persian saying: "I cried because I had no shoes until I met a man who had no feet." Sometimes it takes a moment to look outside of your situation long enough to appreciate what is available to you. Sometimes it takes being with another person who "has no feet" for you to realize that you are truly blessed. Today, make a list of ten ways in which you experience abundance in your life.

— DAY 234 —
DEVELOP SELF-AWARENESS

A good life is not necessarily a life absent of conflict and pain. It is in conflict and pain that you may experience your greatest moments. These are moments of true courage, deep faith, unconditional love, and personal evolution. But it is only with self-awareness and time for reflection that you can maintain that calm center even in the midst of the greatest storm. When I work with clients who wish to develop self-awareness, I give them a question that they must ask themselves every thirty minutes. They set their alarm clock or a reminder on their phone or computer with a note that contains the question "What's happening now?" That causes them to pause, check in with themselves on their feelings, thoughts, and physical state, and observe themselves and their environment. This reduces knee-jerk reactions and habitual responses that interfere with the flow of energy. They begin to know themselves on a deeper level, and as a result they connect to others on a deeper level as well. Today, set an alarm, practice observing yourself through this question, and notice how that changes your ability to be effective and more relaxed.

— DAY 235 —
OPEN SPACE FOR MORE

Your business may be off, or you may be experiencing hardship. These are realities. Expand that reality, and make room for what is possible. If your business is slow, what does this open time allow you to do that you have not been able to do? What issues can you address in this quiet time? If you are experiencing hardship, how might you simplify your life in ways that require less consumption of time, money, or energy? If someone you know is ill, can you give that person the gift of presence, laughter, or witnessing so that they might forget their illness for a while and return to their essential self? If you are feeling overwhelmed, how might you bring joy and quiet into this busy space? If you are afraid, who is your model of courage? Engage these questions today, and apply them as a practice to open space for more possibilities.

— DAY 236 —
BE OF SERVICE

Being of service to another is a nurturing action. It nurtures someone else and nurtures you. In times of stress, nurturing yourself can support your journey. Today, choose to nurture someone in some way, and notice how that gift of care also affects you.

— DAY 237 —
DANCE. SING. TELL A STORY.
LISTEN TO SILENCE.

In many ancestral societies, the healers were the shamans, those human beings who could journey into the cosmos to retrieve wisdom and healing for their communities. If you went to a shaman, complaining of a physical illness or emotional distress, the shaman would ask you one of four questions: When did you stop dancing? When did you stop singing? When did you stop being enthralled by stories? When did you stop listening to the silence? We have lost the childlike qualities of dancing for no reason, singing out loud, and storytelling. Our days are filled with noise that does not allow us to connect to our deepest wishes. Today, dance, sing, tell your story, or listen deeply to someone else's story. And at some point today, allow the silence of a still moment to wash over you and heal your wounds.

DAY 238
FIND COURAGE

Today, ask yourself, "What do I feel is at stake if I fail or succeed?" Write down your answers and review your notes from other days to identify what tips will help you engage your courage and move forward.

– DAY 239 –

WRITE YOUR PERSONAL NARRATIVE

What does it mean to be fully human? It may mean different things to different people at different stages in their lives. As you go through your life, what truly matters to you changes. What may have been terribly important in your twenties is an echo compared with what may be important in your forties. One practice I use with my clients is to have them write their history in sections, and today I'll ask you to do the same. First, write about the first fifteen years of your life, then continue to write about your life in fifteen-year increments. Note what events had the greatest impact on you, regardless of whether they were negative or positive. Set this narrative aside and review it in a few days, and that may help you to notice the threads of beliefs and behaviors that run through your life.

DAY 240
REINVENT YOURSELF

At some points in your life, you will begin to feel an unease that you cannot explain. Oftentimes this is catalyzed by a significant event in your life—a birth, a death, a marriage, a divorce, or a career change. By the time you realize that your priorities have changed, you have already begun the change. Today, take some time to write down your current life priorities. Identifying these will help you make better decisions that support the person you are today.

DAY 241
REMEMBER JOY

To remember in every cell of your body is to touch a past experience that has brought you joy. Don't underestimate joy. It is a powerful experience that you remember on a cellular level. It provides a clue to what makes you happy. Today, remember those moments in your life that have made you smile.

— DAY 242 —
SMILE

When looking to reconnect with that joyful and playful person inside you, simply pay attention to what makes you smile as you move through your day. It means slowing down a bit in order to savor the moments in a way that allows you to sense joy, happiness, or humor. When you feel these, you will automatically smile. That is your clue to what may inspire you, and to what you could be doing now to be happier and to create more meaning in your life. The answer to joy is right there.

— DAY 243 —
PAUSE

Your body is wise. When you are too busy to listen or under duress, your body will send you signals. Your breathing will change and your posture will shift, and if you ignore the signals, you will become ill. By tuning in to your body, especially your breathing, you can remain relaxed, focused, and better able to make decisions.

The most useful technique I share with clients to manage conflict and think strategically in the moment is "pause, breathe, center, respond." It takes about three seconds—the amount of time it takes to pause, take a very deep breath into the belly, hold for a second, exhale completely, and center yourself before responding to a person or an event. Physiologically, this act relaxes the body and the oxygen intake clears the brain. It also creates enough mental space for you to be able to respond thoughtfully, rather than to enter into a habitual reaction. Practice it today.

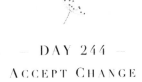

DAY 244
ACCEPT CHANGE

Life is dynamic; it never stops changing. Think of a river that flows constantly. It has its turbulent times and its calm times. You can swim in a river a hundred times, but you'll never swim in the same river more than once. The water has changed, the life in the river has changed, and you have changed. Notice what is changing in your life, and write down ways in which you can get into the flow of it today.

DAY 245

REORIENT YOUR LIFE

You may notice a weariness or tiredness that I describe as being tired from the inside out. You may begin to lose optimism. You may become angry and combative or distant in your relationships. Finally, you may lose faith and hope. These are indications to *stop*! If you do not stop voluntarily, something will happen to make you stop. I have seen this time and time again. These events are powerful, even devastating. They cause you to see yourself essentially, devoid of all the trappings of how you define yourself in the outside world. You get a glimpse of your mortality. You see your impermanence. You begin to see that you are a single drop in a very large ocean. Based on this awareness, take advantage of the opportunity to reorient your life around what really does matter to you now.

DAY 246
ACCEPT THAT YOU ARE MORE

There are days when you feel as if you cannot take one more step. There are days when you are overwhelmed. There are days when you exclaim to no one in particular, "I'm done—I cannot keep going!" Instead of stopping there, consider this a place to rest before you gather up your strength and resolve and continue on your journey. See these days or these moments as an invitation to exceed your limiting beliefs, an invitation to becoming more than you believed you could become. Pause, breathe, then get up and keep walking toward your dreams.

DAY 247
CONNECT TO SPIRIT

Our days are so full of the transactional things that happen in life that we often forget our spiritual nature. Whether you find spirit in quiet contemplation, in a church or synagogue, in nature, or elsewhere, connect today to something that is greater than you. The daily complaints of life will diminish in front of a greater power, and there you will find peace.

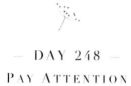

— DAY 248 —
PAY ATTENTION

As you go through your day, notice how you feel. Does something seem to be missing? Look not only for the emptiness but also for those people, events, places, and things that make you smile or relax. These are clues to what makes you happy.

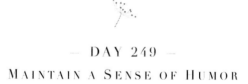

— DAY 249 —
MAINTAIN A SENSE OF HUMOR

As you begin to better manage your life, you will encounter some resistance within yourself and within your environment. Keep a sense of humor about the changes you make. Take things lightly and do things that make you laugh and smile, so that you always uphold your optimism and positive outlook.

— DAY 250 —
ELEVATE YOUR STANDARDS

When you have always measured your happiness by one standard, it becomes difficult to create a new standard. Ask more of yourself and less from the external world. Identify your true measure of happiness. Don't listen to the messages in the media telling you what you need to be happy. You will find that answer within your heart.

— DAY 251 —
LOVE YOURSELF

Everything begins with love. Our struggles are the result of our separation from love. Love is a fountain within you. It is not outside; it is inside. Begin to accept and love yourself. Drink from your own fountain.

— DAY 252 —
BREAK OLD PATTERNS

Old patterns are hard to break. The old patterns will try to reassert themselves when you meet an obstacle. You will think they represent a familiar place to go, but that is not the right place for you any longer. Don't beat yourself up if you falter. Renew your commitment, get back in touch through stillness, and move on.

— DAY 253 —
ENJOY EVOLVING

What you may find in enjoying the evolving you is that there is no "new" you; it is simply that the memory of your essential self has returned to you. You will be more comfortable and happy if you are living by your own values and standards than you would be if you were living by someone else's. The world will open up to you differently than before. You will feel more alive and engaged.

— DAY 254 —
HEED EMERGENCIES

Learn to distinguish true emergencies from false urgencies. You may determine something to be an emergency simply because someone is telling you so. Ask questions first, review your availability, and determine whether a request is really urgent or whether you have access to an alternate response time. Ask first, and then respond thoughtfully.

Overcommitment makes it difficult to deal with real emergencies, so be sure to allow space and time for them. Allocate more than enough resources in terms of support, energy, and time to be able to handle the unexpected without compromising your well-being or your priorities.

— DAY 255 —
REDUCE OVERCOMMITMENT

Have you considered why you always run late or take on too much? Overcommitment has its origins in your self-identity. I have clients who believe they can do it all until they make commitments that they cannot keep or produce sloppy work. Later, they feel badly about it, since their self-identity and ego are strongly rooted in their capacity to work, in their self-reliance, and in their independence. The over-extension of this quality is what drives them to say yes when they should be saying no. Today, determine where you are overcommitting and begin to make space in your life for the unpredictable and for your own self-care.

DAY 256
STAY CENTERED

Learn ways of remaining centered in the midst of great activity or chaos. Everything is constantly changing. The paradox is how to stay still and centered while in motion. Keep a physical reminder on your desk or within your field of vision (an inspirational message, a picture, a candle, a water fountain, a stone you can hold in your hand) that helps you hold your center in the midst of chaos.

DAY 257
PRIORITIZE

You may think that saying no to someone is hurtful or not supportive. If you have trouble using this powerful two-letter word, reframe the response. Ask more questions to determine what is really needed. Delegate the task to someone else, or refer the person to someone else. Create space in which to think about your response by saying, "Let me get back to you on this," or "Let me think about this," or "Let me double-check my availability." Giving yourself time to respond to requests teaches you to break out of the habitual pattern of saying yes to everyone and everything.

DAY 258
BECOME AN ARTIST

Every great masterpiece started with a blank canvas. Stop imitating. Start creating. Pretend that your life is a blank canvas, and create your masterpiece.

— DAY 259 —
DON'T SWEAT THE SMALL STUFF

Assess and eliminate what drains you. Orient around your priorities, and let go of the minor things in life that drain your energy away from focusing on what you want to create.

— DAY 260 —
INTEGRATE THE PAST

When confronted today with a situation like one yesterday, you may gravitate to what has worked in the past, without giving thought to new conditions. Your past does not dictate your future, but by integrating the experiences of your past as if they were lessons, you can become wiser about leading a joyful life. Today, make a note of past experiences that you can view as such lessons.

— DAY 261 —

GET AN OUTSIDE PERSPECTIVE

Sometimes what you think you know is worse than not knowing at all. You may be limited by what you think you know. Getting an outside, objective person to point out your behaviors or to reflect your thought process back to you may be enough to rouse you into more thoughtful patterns.

— DAY 262 —

RELEASE YOUR FEAR OF FAILURE

It may feel safer to you to react in the same manner than to change your reaction. In changing your reactions, you break the existing dynamic. Your fear may be the loss of a relationship, hurting someone's feelings, or making the wrong decision. But failure is failure only if you don't learn from it and move on. Failure is information that you need in order to make adjustments.

— DAY 263 —

CHANGE YOUR HABITS

If you look closely at some of your habitual patterns or responses, you may find that you are avoiding something. As an example, saying "I am tired" may be your response to avoiding conflict or a difficult conversation. One client responded to critiques of her work by diminishing someone else's work. She was unaware that she was doing this but then wondered why her work relationships were tenuous, until we replayed these types of situations word for word. Adapt your language so that you respond thoughtfully and not defensively.

— DAY 264 —

CHOOSE A DIFFERENT RESPONSE

It takes courage and support to break out of habitual responses and patterns. There is always the fear that something more is at stake, but what you stand to lose are really just old, limiting ways of being and stress. Focus on what you stand to *gain* by breaking the habitual cycles you have created.

Innovative solutions, well-being, values-oriented decisions, and life on purpose are the real benefits on the horizon!

— DAY 265 —
CONSIDER SUCCESS

Today, ask yourself, "Am I looking for success, or I am seeking significance?" Define what "success" and "significance" mean to you before you answer.

— DAY 266 —
SEE YOURSELF DIFFERENTLY

We are all stardust, particles of universal energy. We are made of the same stuff as the planets and the stars. The same elements that are found in animals and plants are also in us. Today, consider this meditation—*I am one with all*—and you will begin to see yourself as much more than you ever imagined.

DAY 267
MOVE TOWARD SOMETHING

You may want to create something out of a need to avoid a consequence, or you may want to run away from something that is uncomfortable. You cannot achieve positive results with negative behaviors. Moving away from something is similar to running backward—awkward, difficult, and slow—and you won't get very far. Notice when you are running away from something, and reframe it as a vision of what you want to manifest. Run toward *that* with more energy and ease.

DAY 268
BE OPEN TO POSSIBILITIES

Life takes you where you need to go, not necessarily where you thought you would go. Stay open to possibilities that arrive unannounced and unintended. They are often the ones that hold the greatest potential.

— DAY 269 —
GET A COACH

Anticipate obstacles with the help of a coach, friend, or partner. Create solutions based on your new vision or goal as the focus for your choice. Plan positive solutions in advance of potential obstacles so you are prepared when they arrive.

— DAY 270 —
DEVELOP SUPPORT SYSTEMS

Actively cultivate relationships around you that nudge you into keeping up healthy, productive patterns. Exercise with a friend, post your vision and mission statements, and interact with individuals living on a higher level of consciousness.

— DAY 271 —

MANAGE YOUR FEELINGS

Everything will happen to you. There will be days when things go well and other days when they do not. Remember that, regardless of whether something is positive or negative, this too shall pass. Knowing this will help you maintain a larger perspective and better manage your feelings and emotions.

— DAY 272 —

ACKNOWLEDGE THE PROCESS

Don't beat yourself up if you fall back into old patterns. Recognize that you may be transitioning from one chapter to the next, and that this is all part of the process.

— DAY 273 —
MANAGE YOUR LIFE

Your life is dynamic, and if you are living with attention and intention, you will embrace transitions and shifts with excitement and passion. You can manage your life if you see yourself as the director, not the victim. Transitions will engage you, instead of worrying you. Everyday difficulties will appear less threatening when you see yourself as capable of managing your life. Today, make a note of the areas of your life that you are not managing, and create a plan to get better control of them.

— DAY 274 —
CONNECT TO SOMEONE

Reach out to someone new today. Allow yourself to be a bit vulnerable, and open yourself up to a new friendship. When we protect ourselves, we do not connect with others. The gift behind vulnerability is connection.

— DAY 275 —
SLOW DOWN

To really see and hear, you need to pay attention. In
order to pay attention, you need to slow down. You
need to be still long enough to become fully
present. I often ask my clients to experiment with
walking and talking slowly, or more slowly, as a
practice in presence. Try this today.

— DAY 276 —
CHALLENGE SAFETY

With your mind and with your ego, you develop all
sorts of patterns, habits, and compensating strategies
that help you adapt and succeed with minimum
pain. You are safe. You know your limitations and
excel within those, without venturing too far into
unknown territory. You become adept in your
version of reality. And then one day you wake up.
You see a life, a safe life, but one without passion.
You hunger for evolution but are afraid to step out
into the unknown. "What if?" Today, take a risk

that will challenge your illusion of safety. Speak your opinion in a meeting, post an article on your blog, or volunteer for a new project.

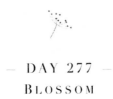

— DAY 277 —
BLOSSOM

Nothing your mind can imagine could possibly be as frightening as flatlining through your life. Your soul knows this. Taking on the "what ifs" requires courage, but the price of not blossoming into your full life is to wither in the snow.

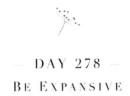

— DAY 278 —
BE EXPANSIVE

Today, ask yourself, "What keeps me from my greatness?" Playing it small and shrinking yourself down helps no one. Share your light.

DAY 279
BECOME A BEGINNER

Do something creative, unusual, and the opposite of what you would "normally" do. Experiment with your life by learning something new. Become a beginner again.

DAY 280
CLEAN OUT THE OLD

Cleaning out the old has not only a physical effect but an emotional effect as well. De-cluttering your home and office serves to create mental space that will allow you to gain new perspectives and re-envision your goals. Take out all that old "garbage," figuratively and literally, to unburden yourself and make room for the new.

— DAY 281 —
SEEK COMMUNITY

Connect with friends, family, and people in your community. In the winter, we tend to hibernate, so we may lose track of our relationships. Have you noticed that you haven't seen your neighbor all season? Write a note or host a party in your neighborhood to catch up.

— DAY 282 —
CHANNEL YOUR ENERGY

Eliminate tolerations and incompletions. Tolerations are things that you put up with that drain your energy. Incompletions are things that hang over you, left undone, and drain you of mental energy. If you are putting up with something, eliminate this energy drain. Choose an alternative, positive channel for this energy.

— DAY 283 —
LIGHTEN UP

Go on a field trip with your kids. Invite your friends over for a potluck dinner. Go for a hike or walk in the woods. Run a race for a favorite charity. Visit the circus. Do something *fun*!

— DAY 284 —
CONQUER NEEDINESS

Where in your life are you feeling needy? Neediness may be sabotaging your efforts to move forward in your life. Is it silently driving you to be a certain way, or to do certain things, that actually keep you from feeling successful or fulfilled? Replace neediness with self-care. When you give yourself what you need or crave, you will replace neediness with confidence. Do something today that you know will build your confidence.

— DAY 285 —
PRACTICE SELF-CARE

The word "selfish" has come to mean something that implies "at the expense of others." Fundamentally, selfishness is care of self without any requirement to do harm to others. Take responsibility for your own self-care by valuing yourself as much as you value others.

— DAY 286 —
CULTIVATE YOUR RELATIONSHIPS

If you are feeling the emptiness of a lost relationship, look to the relationships you enjoy and think about how you might spend more time cultivating those. You may find that doing so leads you to new and energizing relationships.

— DAY 287 —
CHOOSE ABUNDANCE OVER SCARCITY

If a financial crunch and its messages of scarcity are affecting your mood, take another look at what you may have to contribute from your heart, your talents, your hobbies, your time, and elsewhere. These contributions are meaningful, as they reflect your personal gifts to someone else.

— DAY 288 —
FACE YOUR FEAR

We all feel fear at some point, but fear is not "bad"; in fact, it can be useful. It indicates that there is something present to which we must pay attention. Courage is the constructive engagement of fear. Think of a thing you have been afraid of, or an activity you have been afraid of doing. Write down specifically what frightens you about it. Then creatively find ways to engage the fear, perhaps through research, perhaps by talking to someone who has gone through the same thing, or perhaps by challenging assumptions you may be making. You will find that fear can be an ally in creating your life and your work.

— DAY 289 —
FIVE DAYS OF QUESTIONS

For the next five days, I will ask questions that can provide direction toward where you want to go, starting with where you have been. These questions are designed for you to take stock of where you are in your life and to begin to create a vision of a new way of managing and living your life. Today, begin to assess your current reality, and write down the vision of the life you want.

DAY 290
FIVE DAYS OF QUESTIONS:
ACCOMPLISHMENT

Today, ask yourself, "What do I feel are my greatest accomplishments? What helped me achieve them?" Be sure to record these in your journal, and look for clues about what creates the flow of energy to achieve. Frequently look back on your accomplishments to maintain a sense of success.

DAY 291
FIVE DAYS OF QUESTIONS:
CHALLENGES

There will be days when you feel as if the challenges are greater than the rewards. What are your current challenges? What is getting in the way of your having the life you want? Record your responses, and begin to list options to overcome those challenges and obstacles.

— DAY 292 —

FIVE DAYS OF QUESTIONS:
HIDDEN OPPORTUNITIES

What if the life you really want is hidden behind the problem or chaos you are facing right now? Let me tell you a story. In 2007, I lost the house of my dreams after living in it for only one year. I used to sit on the stairs overlooking the entry and feel so happy that I had finally been able to achieve this goal of having a beautiful home. I was completely shattered when I lost it because of job loss and a failing economy. Years later, I was able to see that beautiful house as an albatross, one that would have kept me prisoner to a mortgage and lifestyle that denied my freedom. Hidden behind this loss was a treasure that I could not see at the time but now appreciate. Take heart: behind what we see as a problem or tragedy is a door to hidden opportunity. Seek it out.

— DAY 293 —
FIVE DAYS OF QUESTIONS:
LIVING WELL

What do you consider a life well lived? Today, give put some distance between yourself and your life, and look for those moments when you shone like a bright light for yourself and others. You were living well, and you continue to do so each time you align with what is true for you.

— DAY 294 —
FIVE DAYS OF QUESTIONS:
COMPLETIONS

Where do you feel incomplete in your relationships, in your work, and/or at home? These areas of incompleteness silently drain you of energy, quietly gnawing at your vitality as you attempt to create a joy-filled life. Write down those things you think are incomplete, and schedule activities to handle them. You will feel more joy and less stress immediately.

— DAY 295 —
PAUSE TO SAY THANK YOU

You have so much to be thankful for, yet chances are that you have not intentionally expressed thanks. Examples include relationships, a comfortable bed, and food on the table. Give thanks, tell those you love that you love them, follow through with actions, and share your good fortune with others.

— DAY 296 —
HANDLE SETBACKS

Everyone encounters setbacks. The key to a successful life is to keep moving past those setbacks and to look at them from a perspective of learning, not failure. The only true failure consists of remaining identified with a perceived failure and not using it as an impetus to do better next time.

— DAY 297 —
LEARN FROM MISTAKES

When working with clients who are stuck in the past and tied to a mistake they made, I use this technique: *Name it. Claim it. Reframe it.* First, identify what happened without blame. Then acknowledge your role in the event. Lastly, create a new interpretation that moves you forward with new learning and motivation.

— DAY 298 —
MAKE A CHANGE

What, if anything, is the major change you need to make in order to realize a dream you have? How are you planning to make that change so that your dream manifests? Typically, there is one fundamental step that is the pivot point for a change. It could be making a decision to go to bed earlier, so that you can get up early to work out and become healthier. Or it could be meeting with a financial advisor to get your finances in order so you can retire well. Identify the major change and the first step you need to take to make your dreams come true.

— DAY 298 —

DEFINE WHAT MATTERS

Take some quiet time to define what is really important to you. How will you arrange your life accordingly? When you can define what really matters, you can start to align with your values to create a joyful and meaningful existence.

— DAY 300 —

GO HOME

Returning home can be a way of connecting to your roots. The food you eat, the way it is cooked, the music that is played, and the generations of people who may gather give you a sense of both roots and familial evolution. It is a place where you welcome the old, young, and new. Gather to celebrate the connection and to give thanks for all that means, or to heal old wounds as you move forward in your life.

DAY 301
SACRIFICE YOUR LIFE

Although the word "sacrifice" implies pain and discomfort, its true meaning is very different. Essentially, "to sacrifice" means "to make sacred." I'm not talking about the small sacrifices of everyday existence; I'm talking about living a spiritual life. From this perspective, begin to view your life as sacred, and you will then view all life as sacred. You are here in this life because you were meant to be here, in order to learn the most profound lesson—the lesson of love. Carry a sense of sacredness with you today and every day, and notice how your life begins to feel and look from that perspective. Your life will truly change when you make it sacred.

DAY 302
TAKE RESPONSIBILITY FOR YOUR LIFE

Don't play the victim. It is your life, and no one else is responsible for it. Only you are responsible for what you do with it, so choose wisely.

DAY 303
VALUE FAMILY TIME

Today's busy families are hard pressed to have meals together or engage in meaningful conversations. In the past, families had traditions and rituals that were specific to them or to their community. What rituals does your family enjoy? How will they create memories for your children? Get together with your family today, and agree on what traditions and rituals your family would like to incorporate every day and on special occasions.

DAY 304
FORGET PERFECTION

Resist pressure to be perfect. Allow for some flexibility and spontaneity. Your family dinner doesn't have to be perfect. Focus on enjoying the relationships, instead of doing the dishes.

— DAY 305 —
HONOR GRIEF AND LOSS

Our culture deals poorly with loss and grief. If you or someone you know has lost someone, be gentle with yourself or with that person today.

— DAY 306 —
CELEBRATE HOLIDAYS

Focus on the true meaning of holidays, whether it's a birthday, an anniversary, or a national or religious holiday. What do these special days mean to you spiritually? Reconnect with that meaning.

— DAY 307 —
PRACTICE UNDERCOMMITTING

Don't overcommit yourself or make promises you know you cannot keep. First, make time for yourself and those who really matter to you. The rest is optional.

— DAY 308 —
BE A KID AGAIN

I love watching my son when he encounters something new, like a simple campout under the stars in Maine. He has always been full of awe and wonder, and I have been only too happy to join him in that. Play, laugh, and incorporate what you loved as a child. Make memories with your own children.

— DAY 309 —
DISCOVER BREAKTHROUGHS

On the other side of any breakdown is a breakthrough waiting to be discovered. When we experience breakdowns or losses, it's difficult to see the possibility that is hidden there. I remember working myself to exhaustion in my late twenties. I thought that was what a dedicated professional did—until I ended up having a short stay in the hospital, believing that I would lose my job and that the project I was working on would surely fail. What I realized was that I was surrounded by competent people who could take care of the project while I took care of myself. I got some much-needed rest, and returned renewed and with a deeper appreciation for my coworkers. That was my breakthrough.

— DAY 310 —
SHARE GOOD FEELINGS

Be sure to take time to appreciate the good in your life today and to share this with others. When you share goodness, you add positive energy to others' lives, too.

— DAY 311 —
DON'T OVERDO IT

Eat healthfully and get plenty of sleep—and if you have time off, extra cuddling is especially nice on wintry mornings!

— DAY 312 —

ESTABLISH MOMENTUM

Do you want to accomplish something? Be present in the moment-to-moment. It's the very definition of "momentum"!

— DAY 313 —

SEE THE PLUSES AND MINUSES IN EVERYTHING

We always have a choice to see the positive in the negative or the negative in the positive. Don't get hung up on one or the other. Both serve a purpose.

— DAY 314 —

STAY OR CHANGE COURSE APPROPRIATELY

Very little in life is permanent, so keep that perspective as you make decisions and choices. Most of the time, you will be able to change course or change your mind. Don't let one decision dictate the rest of your life.

— DAY 315 —
ACCEPT THAT LIFE IS EVER-CHANGING

Life can be difficult, but struggle is optional. Struggle happens when you resist what is present and right in front of you. When you want things to be what they are not, you struggle. Accept what is, and from that acceptance begin to generate what you need.

— DAY 316 —
CHANGE YOUR BEHAVIOR
AND YOUR STORY

Does changing your behavior change your story, or does changing your story change your behavior? The answer: yes. It doesn't matter. What matters is to recognize the behavior and the story, and then choose how and what you will change and how that will help you be more successful and happy.

DAY 317

BECOME AN ASTRONAUT

When I was little, I wanted to be an astronaut. I would gaze up into the sky and wonder what it would be like to explore space. That wonderment was the seed of curiosity and imagination that I still have inside me. It doesn't matter whether your dream is realistic sometimes; what matters is that you maintain a sense of wonder and possibility in a world that at times seems hostile to dreams.

DAY 318

BEWARE OF ALL THAT GLITTERS

You will be seduced—by people, money, or status; by your desire to fit in; even by your own goals and dreams. Always keep someone near to you who is a truthsayer, someone or something that will always reflect your true Self back to you, that can be your compass when you lose your way. The world will try to change you, often with good intentions. Happiness is born of an authentic life. Be who you are, and at the same time know that who you are will evolve. Pay attention to your heart and soul. The heart, not the mind, is the true sage.

— DAY 319 —
WRITE IT DOWN

Today, ask yourself, "Am I managing my life, or is life managing me? What's working? What's not working?" Now, start writing what needs to change so you can better manage what's not working and make more time for what is.

— DAY 320 —
EMBRACE THE UNKNOWN

There is no adventure in certainty. If you are looking for safety or security, or if you think you know the future, you will experience stress and disappointment. Life is an adventure, and you never know what you will find around the next corner.

— DAY 321 —
EXPERIMENT WITH LIFE

Life can be an experiment in happiness if you are willing to lose your unhappiness. Some people are attached to their unhappiness. Be the person who claims your happy place, and see what results from your new attitude.

— DAY 322 —
TAKE YOUR TIME

If you want to be someone who enjoys life, then you may want to look at everything you do and ask: Which activities contribute to your life and which ones detract from the life you really want? You can't get to "be" through "do." Sometimes you need to stop "doing" so you can just "be."

— DAY 323 —
MANIFEST YOUR GREATNESS

Happiness comes with the alignment of your values and your actions. What you care about becomes manifest in your life. Let your values and what you care about be the criteria you use when you make decisions about your life.

— DAY 324 —
LEARN HOW TO TALK WITH YOUR HEART

Matthias Mehl, a psychologist at the University of Arizona, found that people who engaged in substantive conversations actually experienced more happiness than those who spent most of their time in superficial conversations. He attributed this finding to two main causes: 1) human beings are driven to find and create meaning in their lives, and 2) humans need to connect with other people. When you engage someone in conversation today, make it count. Speak from the heart, and share that happiness with someone else.

DAY 325
PRACTICE ACCEPTANCE

Today, ask yourself, "What part of my self am I not accepting?" We all have those disowned parts of us that we carry around in the shadows. To begin to accept these in yourself is also to accept flaws in others. Acceptance brings peace and wholeness to you and to your relationships.

DAY 326
DON'T BUY HAPPINESS

You know the feeling: you go out to window-shop and come back with bags of new clothes, shoes, and whatever else caught your attention. Suddenly, the savings you were going to use to see your family or to explore some part of the world have leaked into shopping malls and boutiques. Although these things make you happy for the moment, consider the trade-off. Like someone who binges on ice cream to appease an emotional need, you may be doing the same with shopping. Today, take a moment to consider where your money should and should not go. Make a conscious decision to use your money for what really matters.

DAY 327
CONNECT TO YOUR WISDOM

Think about a time when you felt confident in yourself, able to meet a challenge because you really knew what was true for you, maybe even despite evidence to the contrary. That is your greater wisdom speaking to you. What does that feel like? Choose a current situation and apply this wisdom to the situation. Practice wisdom.

DAY 328
SHARE HAPPY

Everyone deserves someone to share "happy" with. Look for healthy relationships that align with what you care about. A healthy relationship allows each person to share his or her happiness with gratitude.

— DAY 329 —
ENJOY THE VIEW

A few years ago, a friend of mine talked me into going rock climbing. It was only a rock wall at a spa, but the experience was unforgettable. After watching several people struggle to climb the wall, I surprised myself by making it to the top in the shortest amount of time. The whole time, I never looked away from the wall. I had started to ready myself to rappel down, when the instructor told me to stop and look around. Poised at the top, I looked around. I was in Arizona and high enough to see the sun lighting the desert with hues of pinks and purples. It was a stunning view that I would have missed in pursuit of my task. My lesson: Don't forget to pause to experience happiness while you are in pursuit of it. Drink in the view.

— DAY 330 —
SAY YES OR SAY NO

When you say yes to something, you say no to something else. When you say no to something, you say yes to something else. Usually, you are saying yes or no to yourself. Your time and energy are valuable. Choose your commitments wisely to better manage your life.

— DAY 331 —
CHERISH LOVE

Never take love for granted. When you take love for granted by assuming that it will always be there, that it will always grow, that it needs no attention—that is when you will lose it. Love needs love. Like any living thing, love needs to be nurtured, acknowledged, and acted upon. Revel in true love. It is God's greatest gift.

— DAY 332 —

BE A GOOD AND TRUSTWORTHY FRIEND

Friends keep you sane in times of trouble. True friends are there in the darkest moments with no conditions or judgments. They are there in the joyous moments, too, celebrating life with you. Be a good friend, and you will attract good friends. Never sacrifice yourself for others—true friends make no such demands. They will love you for exactly who you are.

— DAY 333 —

THINK HOLISTICALLY

There is more to life than struggle. Think holistically. What areas of your life are going well and what are the areas where you experience struggle? Could the energy you expend in struggle be channeled into more meaningful endeavors? Remind yourself that each time you struggle is a call to pay attention and an opportunity to be strong and to transform that energy into something constructive.

— DAY 334 —

S*#T HAPPENS, AND SO DOES GRACE

One winter morning, my dog, Finn, woke me at six thirty, needing to go outside. Anyone who knows me knows I am not a morning person. Grumpily, I got up, slipped on my robe and a pair of shoes, and took him outside into the chilly morning. As he was doing his business, I began to feel the cool air and to listen to the multitude of birdsongs as the sun rose through the trees. I began to breathe in the dewy air, and felt the earth's energy waking up. I was in a state of grace at the same moment that "s*#t" was happening, literally. Isn't that life, though? S*#t happens, and we can still choose grace!

— DAY 335 —

STAY UP LATE

There are times I can't sleep when I surrender to the sleeplessness by taking a walk outside. The first few times I did this, I heard sounds that I didn't recognize, those of all kinds of night creatures reveling in the darkness. There is so much we don't know because we have yet to experience all of life. Do something you don't normally do, and notice what becomes alive in you. Stay up late. Listen to the night songs. They are there for you to hear if you are paying attention. Listen.

— DAY 336 —
CALL A FRIEND TODAY

What does friendship mean to you? Do you know who will still be standing alongside you ten years from now? The longest I have known someone who is currently in my life, aside from family members, is a woman named Maria. After a couple of years of losing track of each other, we reconnected. I have known her since I was fifteen! Each time we talk, it is as if no time has passed, yet we still learn something new about each other. Are there people like this in your life? Appreciate them. They are rare gems. Call them today.

— DAY 337 —
STAY OPEN IN HARDSHIP

Do not harden yourself in the face of loss and betrayal. Sorrow and grief can become imprisoned inside us through the hardening and armoring that we use to defend our tender places. Learn to move with the turbulent currents of life, not against them, and your losses and betrayals will not consume or break you.

— DAY 338 —
BECOME AN ALCHEMIST

Your best friends are those people who have walked through the fire with you. There is a kind of alchemy that occurs in friendships forged by sharing history, both good times and difficult times. Through your friends, you become more than you thought you could be. They see all the parts of you, even the ones you would like to hide, yet your best friends remain in your life. The alchemy between friends allows you to forge the bonds that always sustain you. Notice this alchemy happening next time you are in conversation with good friends. It will make you smile.

— DAY 339 —
RECOVER MEMORIES

I have an uncanny memory for what can appear to be personal trivia. I remember the names of kids in kindergarten that I used to play with. I remember phone numbers, including the phone number of the first house I lived in as a child. I remember who gave me gifts I received years ago. I have realized that the reason I remember these innocuous things is that I associate some emotion or feeling with them. Indeed, what I am remembering is that emotion or feeling. What do you remember, and why?

— DAY 340 —
TAP INTO YOUR SENSES

Your senses are keepers of memories that your mind may have forgotten. One of the strongest senses is the olfactory. The smell of newly-mown grass never ceases to elicit memories of my father mowing the lawn as we all helped him with yard work. That memory grounds me. What personal memories do you associate with smells and scents? Today, begin to identify how you can tap your senses to bring about a sense of well-being and happiness at any moment.

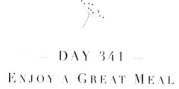

— DAY 341 —
ENJOY A GREAT MEAL

Billions of dollars are spent each year on dieting and diet products and services. That makes me question our relationship to food. What is it that you really want to control when you diet? Why has food become the enemy, something to conquer? I still associate certain foods and meals with building connections between friends and family, and I refuse to give that up for the sake of caloric management. Today, begin to change your personal relationship with food in order to see it as nurturing and providing vitality.

– DAY 342 –
FIND ENJOYMENT IN EXERCISE

I hate to exercise. As disciplined as I am in other areas of my life, I dislike physical effort because I dislike physical discomfort. I know I am not alone. Yet I do exercise. I have had to reframe it as activities I enjoy—like biking, kayaking, walking, and yoga, in addition to traditional strength training—that also keep me healthy. If you hate exercise, identify your own ways to reframe it so that you can find enjoyment, as well as health.

– DAY 343 –
SET ASIDE YOUR JUDGMENTS

Witnessing means being completely present, without judgment or comment, to another person's struggle, victory, confusion, enlightenment, joy, thoughts, and feelings. It means that you set aside your own ego and assumptions. Who in your life or work needs a witness? Can you provide that for them? Who is your compassionate witness? Play that part for someone else today.

— DAY 344 —

LEARN, AND THEN LEARN MORE

Learning is vastly different from knowing, yet I see them confused all the time. In schools, as in organizations, individuals are rewarded for knowing, not learning. Learning takes curiosity and risk. Knowing is limiting. The most successful individuals are those who are curious about what they don't know and willing to step into uncertainty in order to learn. Choose something you would like to learn about, get curious, and learn something totally new today.

— DAY 345 —

NOTICE YOUR DEFAULT PATTERNS

We all have our default mechanisms. This is where we go when we are under stress, afraid, and reactive. We stay in our comfort zones or we default to old patterns of thinking and behaving that may no longer be successful. What could you be doing differently in order to get the results you want in life and in work? Notice what your default patterns are.

DAY 346
LOVE DOGS

I have had four dogs in my life. Each one has contributed something very special. Each one has been a teacher to me. Dogs have a way of wriggling into your heart in a way that no other creature can do. In the next six days, I will share my lessons from dogs. These lessons hold true wisdom.

DAY 347
LESSONS FROM DOGS, #1

If you want to learn presence, get a dog.

DAY 348
LESSONS FROM DOGS, #2

If you want to be joyful, watch a dog at play.

DAY 349
LESSONS FROM DOGS, #3

If you want to know peace, watch a dog nap.

DAY 350
LESSONS FROM DOGS, #4

If you want to learn unconditional love, come home to a dog.

DAY 351
LESSONS FROM DOGS, #5

If you want to see someone who is fully alive, take a dog on a car ride and let him stick his head out the window as he savors the wind.

— DAY 352 —

LESSONS FROM DOGS, #6

If you want to know what loyalty is, get sick and notice your dog next to you for days as you heal.

— DAY 353 —

LESSONS FROM CATS

For all you cat lovers, if you want to learn true, unabashed relaxation, get a cat; they feel just purr-fect lying lazily in a sunny window, pretending not to care about the world passing by.

— DAY 354 —

ACKNOWLEDGE YOUR CONNECTION TO ALL THINGS

One of the most life-changing things I've ever done was to go tracking with my friend Paul Rezendes in the Berkshires many years ago. From Paul, I experienced how interconnected living things are. How might you behave if you lived as if you were connected to all living beings? Today, look around your world and see yourself this way.

— DAY 355 —
ENJOY SOLITUDE

Have you ever spent a week all by yourself, with no input from the modern world? Have you taken the time to be in a cabin in the mountains or in a cottage by the ocean, with no computer, radio, TV, or Internet? Try this sometime, and bring your journal. There's no telling what you may discover in the silence of nature.

— DAY 356 —
UNDERSTAND YOUR TRUE NATURE

What if you don't know the answer to the question "Who am I"? What then? How can you connect with the essence of who you are, instead of the outer face you show to the world? Think about your childhood, before society's norms and rules inhibited you. What did you enjoy? Play is another way to recover your true nature. Incorporate playfulness and lightness into your life, into your language, and into your work, and you will begin to see your true nature emerge.

— DAY 357 —
RISE AND SHINE

Each morning this week, pause before you rise from bed, and scan your body. Does it feel rested, tense, tired, or energized? Is that how you want to feel? Start a ritual the evening before that allows you to rise the way you want to feel. You may decide to go to bed earlier or to eat a lighter dinner or to sit quietly before bed. Rest before sleep, and your sleep will improve.

— DAY 358 —
STROLL IN THE SUNRISE
OR THE MOONLIGHT

If you are a night person, try rising early in the morning and connect with that morning energy when the world is waking up, with all its chatter and dew and new sun. If you are a morning person, try staying up late and, if the weather is appropriate, take a stroll in the moonlight to connect with the receptive lunar energy of the night.

— DAY 359 —
CLEAN OUT YOUR CLOSET

Cleaning out my closet is almost a meditative practice for me. I have a two-year rule: if I haven't worn it in two years, it is donated. This ritual allows me to de-clutter, physically and mentally, and to decide on purpose what I keep and what goes—and this translates into other areas of my life as well. Clean out your closets or garage this week, recycle or donate, and make way for fresh energy to enter.

— DAY 360 —
PRACTICE GRATITUDE

For the next five days, I will give you specific practices in gratitude. I believe that we do not practice gratitude enough. The rewards of these practices are abundance and well-being. Get ready to practice. Today, begin by thinking about what gratitude means to you.

— DAY 361 —
GRATITUDE PRACTICE #1

Pick three relationships you are grateful for. Tell these people that you appreciate them, and why.

— DAY 362 —
GRATITUDE PRACTICE #2

Pick three physical things you are grateful for (your home, a favorite book, your yoga mat), and notice the reason they mean something to you.

DAY 363
GRATITUDE PRACTICE #3

Pick three friends whom you haven't seen in a long time. Call them and reconnect; tell them why they are still in your thoughts and your heart.

DAY 364
GRATITUDE PRACTICE #4

Pick three mentors, guides, or teachers from your past and tell them how they have affected your life.

DAY 365
GRATITUDE PRACTICE #5

Create a prayer of gratitude that you can say every morning or evening in order to create mindfulness around the abundance in your life. When things are difficult, this prayer or meditation will buoy you and remind you that even in scarce times, there is abundance.

One Year, 365 Days Later

I hope you have enjoyed *Manage Your Life Before Life Manages You*. By now you have incorporated more joy and less stress. You have learned much about yourself on the way. You have inquired into your beliefs and made shifts in your thinking, and you are taking new, more productive actions toward creating a life designed around what matters most to you. You can repeat these practices every year, and each year the results will be slightly different for you. You will notice how you have grown and evolved as a human being.

If you'd like additional support, please contact me for help on next steps. Stay in touch by signing up for my newsletter, following my blog and my Facebook page, and checking me out on Twitter @aliciarod. If you have any comments, please e-mail me at Alicia@boldconversations.com.

All of my contact information appears at the end of the book.

> With gratitude to you, my dear reader,
> Alicia

EXERCISES AND RESOURCES

In the section that follows, I've included some reflective questions, coaching exercises, thoughtful frameworks, and development models that I use with my clients. Working with these will provide deeper insight into how to make adjustments so that you can create a life in alignment with what you value, as well as creating more joy and ease. Take your time with these exercises, and if you would like additional support, you can contact me through:

www.boldconversations.com

My best wishes for
your continued success.

CLIENT EXERCISE: BIG QUESTIONS

Be thoughtful about your responses to the questions below. You may want to complete some, and then come back to it to complete it later as you reflect on your answers.

BIG PICTURE

If a coach could be a magic lamp, what would happen when you rubbed it?

What's most important to you: values, goals, or states of being?

Obstacles

What's holding you back?

Are you satisfied with your life as it is now?

If you are called to something more, what is it?

Do you have any messes to clean up or incompletions draining your cup?

What are you putting up with or merely tolerating that's holding you back?

Do you have enough time for what is important to you?

LIFE PURPOSE; WORK

Do you feel like your life has a purpose, an aim? What is it?

Is it important to you to have a purpose?

Does your work satisfy you?

Is anything missing?

Relationships

Do you need people/community?

Do you need solitude/quiet time?

Are you satisfied with your relationships with people?

Do you want something else, more, less, in your relationships? What?

Are you satisfied with your relationship with yourself?

Do you want something else, more, less? What?

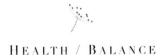

HEALTH / BALANCE

How is your health/energy/vitality?

Do you take care of yourself?

Is anything missing?

How do you enjoy yourself? (Recreation, fun, inspiration . . .)

Is a spiritual life, however you define it, important to you?

How would you describe it?

Action

What is the possibility you want to create?

What part of you is calling to be expressed yet is not currently being expressed?

What has to change in order for you to live a life that reflects what matters to you the most? Identify three things:

1.

2.

3.

What's the BIG CHANGE?

If you were to change these things, how would your life be different/improved?

1.

2.

3.

4.

5.

(More?)

What is the first step to take in the direction of the change you identified?

How would you like to be, or need to be, coached?

Name: ....

Telephone Number: ....

E-mail: ....

Date: ....

Send this to your coach.

AVOID-CREATE MODEL

Which way are you approaching your situation or challenge? Use a situation in your life right now that is challenging you to determine if you are avoiding something or creating something. You move toward what you focus on!

PROCESS OF AVOIDANCE	PROCESS OF CREATION
Is energy being funneled into avoiding something?	Is energy being funneled into creating something?
Movement: Avoiding mistakes of the past	Movement: Creating what you want in the future
Emotion: Fear	Emotion: Hope
Energy: Negative	Energy: Positive

Flow: Effortful	Flow: Effortless
Direction: Moving away from	Direction: Being drawn toward
Sensation: Heavy	Sensation: Lightness
Other: Worry	Other: Energy

MY PERSONAL MANDALA

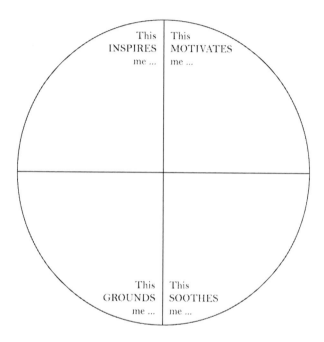

This
INSPIRES
me ...

This
MOTIVATES
me ...

This
GROUNDS
me ...

This
SOOTHES
me ...

Complete your personal mandala. In each quadrant, write what inspires, motivates, grounds, and soothes you.

My Personal Mantra:

My Personal Theme Song:

What throws me off center?

What gets me back to center?

How present is this in my life and work?

How can I include it or access it at any moment?

As I look at my mandala, which area needs more attention?

What can I tell myself or others about caring for the self?

What is missing that I need to include?

Self-Awareness/Resiliency Exercise

What are the top five "needs"—or, a better way of saying it, "requirements for well-being"—that must be met in order for you to decrease your stress and increase your capacity to handle changes at work (example: quiet time for self)?

1.

2.

3.

4.

5.

What is the request that you could make to get each of these needs addressed/met? And to whom will you make the request?

1.

2.

3.

4.

5.

What are the first, second, and third actions you need to take to get these needs addressed/met?

1.

2.

3.

What is the effect you will experience once these needs/requirements are met?

1.

2.

3.

4.

5.

How will the effect of getting these needs/require-
ments met impact your ability to lead your staff,
manage yourself, and effectively handle changes at
work?

1.

2.

3.

4.

5.

Anything else—other comments, insights?

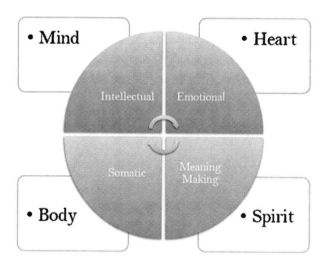

Everyone, especially women, must learn to pay attention to the four quadrants of their lives, which comprise a unified wellness approach to life. These quadrants are The Mind (Intellectual), The Body (Somatic), The Heart (Emotional), and most importantly, The Spiritual (Meaning-Making). Explore how these areas are nourished or deficient in your life. By harmonizing these aspects, you are able to tap Power and Presence.

Here is a reflective exercise for you:

Question: "What contributes to my power and presence in the middle of everything that is coming at me all day long? How can I stay grounded even as chaos swirls around me?

Answer: "You must have a sense of yourself that is *spacious enough* to handle whatever arises. Breathe and create space."

SHOULDS EXERCISE

What you believe you should have or do or be will keep you from being authentic and ultimately happy with yourself and your life. This exercise will reveal what you believe about yourself and how that creates "shoulds" that keep you from being fully present in your life. Do this exercise honestly and in silence allowing the truth to come through. You may discover that you are creating a story that is solely based in fear not reality.

THE SHOULDS I HAVE/DO	WHAT IF I DIDN'T...	THEN....
EX: I _should_ make a lot of money.	I would be a failure.	I would be a bag lady.

A WISDOM PRACTICE: PAUSE, BREATHE, CENTER, RESPOND (PBCR)

Here is a practice I give to my clients that I also practice in times of stress. This could be when conflict arises, when something unpredictable occurs, or when I am tired. This practice can apply to many situations—where it works best is within stressful situations, situations that require clear thinking, situations that deal with conflict, or when you are moving quickly from one task to another.

It is *"Pause, Breathe, Center, Respond."*

It takes about three seconds—the amount of time it takes to pause, take a very deep breath in all the way down into your belly, hold for a second, exhale completely, and come back to one's inner center asking yourself, "What do I want from this interaction?" or "What is my most effective response or action?" and from that place respond to the person or to the event. Physiologically, it moves you out of the Fight or Flight response that depletes your thinking brain of oxygen, it relaxes the body and relieves tension, and it provides the oxygen intake that clears the brain. It also creates enough space (in the pause) to be able to respond thoughtfully rather than to enter into a habitual reaction.

Here is an example: "Mary" was presenting to her directors on a new marketing plan. After presenting, one senior manager attacked the plan and attempted to provoke her into a reactionary response. She did not respond immediately even though she felt personally attacked. Instead, she quietly paused, breathed, and centered herself, and she was able to respond with great clarity and confidence, without any acrimony or defensiveness. Her plan was approved.

Another example: "Mike" moves quickly in his day from meeting to meeting to the point that he was losing track of what he wanted to actually accomplish in each meeting. By the end of the day, he was exhausted and feeling as if he had not accomplished anything. By practicing the four-part PBCR between meetings, he was able to complete his thinking on one meeting, pause, and shift to focus on the desired outcome of the following meeting. He was more productive, more engaged in each meeting, made better decisions, communicated more effectively, and felt energized, not drained, by the pace of his day.

As you go through your day, practice P-B-C-R. It will allow you to remain focused, it will keep you from habitual responses that do not have positive results, and it will maintain wellness in your body as well as your mind.

Now: Pause – Breathe – Center – Respond

REMOVE ENERGY DRAINS

Because of habit or a lack of attention, we keep people, things, events, and habits in our life that drain our energy. Maybe you have not yet completed your taxes and the deadline is looming, or you have not made an appointment with your doctor for a yearly check up. Perhaps your car needs a tune up and the constant rattling is beginning to wear on your nerves. These are things that you tolerate, yet they silently drain your energy.

Make a list of these tolerations.

Next to the item, write ideas on ridding yourself of whatever it is you are putting up with.

Toleration Item	Possible Solutions

REFLECTIVE NOTES

ACKNOWLEDGMENTS

Each time I sat down to write a book, I began with the enthusiasm of a child about to play her favorite game. The anticipation of the end result provided inspiration and motivation even when life—with all its details, schedules, and agendas—intruded.

Then there were the moments when doubt crept in, when my inner critic attacked, telling me that no one would care if I ever wrote another word and that writing a book is a hedonistic, self-indulgent activity with no real reward, except for the satisfaction of emptying my brain of useless information. Self-flagellation was allowed and even encouraged in these moments.

Those were the times when I was lucky enough to have a few great friends around to slap me silly and tell me that indeed my thoughts matter and my ideas help others, and that I needed to sit my butt down and continue. For those people, I wish to express my appreciation, thanks, and gratitude.

First and foremost, I want to acknowledge my clients, all the individuals who have had the courage to engage in conversations, to explore their lives in order to make them better, and to create meaning for their existence and work. My clients are the reason I wrote this book. Noticing how stressful life can be and devising practices to increase the joyful moments and decrease the anxious moments has been my work for many years. Without my clients to mirror my own development, I wonder if I would still be the immature young woman who, joyfully but clueless, skipped through life. I prefer the ripeness of age and experience that brings the wisdom held in these pages.

When we enter life, we arrive alone, naked and screaming. The release from the womb is terrifying and a prologue to the life that awaits us. That life is made better when you have a friend or a partner, someone to whom you can turn for comfort, advice, and support. In my life, there have been several individuals who filled that role. I thank all of them. Right now there is a person who has in the past few years been my teacher, mentor, lover, partner, advocate, and inspiration. He has pushed me to the creative edge on a spiritual journey that keeps me standing on the precipice, wanting to leap but still evolving to the point where I could fly. His patience is admirable. To the Happy Shaman, my deepest gratitude and love.

I want to thank Annie Tucker, my editor, for showing me that the experience of editing a book does not have to be the same as lying on a bed of nails or going to the dentist's office. Annie's frank but gentle suggestions have made this book so much better and more useful to you, the reader. My gratitude and continued appreciation, Annie.

And I want to thank you, dear reader, for caring enough about yourself to pick up this book and engage in a daily practice of self-inquiry, self-discovery, and personal evolution. I know these practices work, as I have seen them work with my clients. Thank you for your continued support.

With love,
Alicia

About the Author

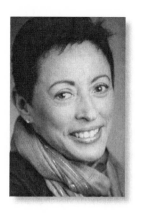

Alicia M. Rodriguez:
Writer. Storyteller. Catalyst.

Alicia is a transformational teacher, leadership advisor, and guide. She inspires and empowers individuals to lead powerfully, live authentically, and act purposefully. She is a dynamic speaker, author, blogger, writer, and visionary whose work unites the world of business with wisdom, mindfulness, and spirituality. She works with leaders from the worlds of business, nonprofit, and social entrepreneurship. Her experience includes powerful strategies in leadership, business, personal, and spiritual development. Ms. Rodriguez is known for her intuition as much as for her results in coaching leaders and individuals who commit to developing themselves from the inside out. The base of her own wisdom lies in her studies of spiritual teachings, psychological frameworks, cognitive science studies, and ancestral wisdom traditions. Alicia lives on the Chesapeake Bay, where she engages her passion for kayaking and writing, and spends part of her time in Ecuador, where she writes and runs a small guest-house and retreat center.

To connect with Alicia,
visit her at any of the following:

www.aliciamrodriguez.com
www.boldconversations.com
www.sophia-associates.com

E-mail: Alicia@aliciamrodriguez.com
Blog: www.boldconversations.com/blog/
Twitter: https://twitter.com/aliciarod
Facebook: https://www.facebook.com/
BoldConversationsBlog

CPSIA information can be obtained at www.ICGtesting.com
Printed in the USA
BVOW02s2010181115

427675BV00001B/1/P